A Guide
to
Homoeopathy

Published by :
Lotus Press Publishers & Distributors

A Guide to Homoeopathy

Dr. Rajeev Sharma
M.D., D.Lit.

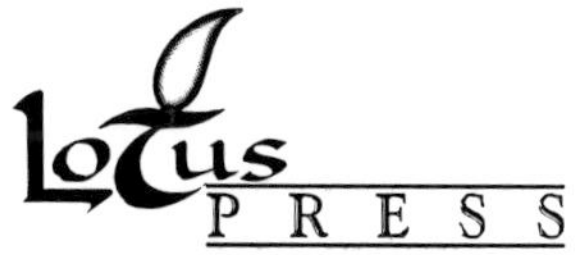

4735/22, Prakash Deep Building
Ansari Road, Darya Ganj,
New Delhi - 110002

Lotus Press : Publishers & Distributors
Unit No. 220, 2nd Floor, 4735/22, Prakash Deep Building,
Ansari Road, Darya Ganj, New Delhi- 110002
Ph.: 23280047, 98118-38000
• E-mail : lotuspress1984@gmail.com
www.lotuspress.co.in

A Guide to Homoeopathy

ISBN: 81-8382-116-2

Attention Readers:
Every effort is made to ensure accuracy of material, but the publisher, printer and author will not be held responsible for any inadvertent error(s). In case of any dispute, all legal matters to be settled under Delhi Jurisdiction only.

Printed & Published by : **Lotus Press Publishers & Distributors,** New Delhi-02

Dr. Rajeev Sharma

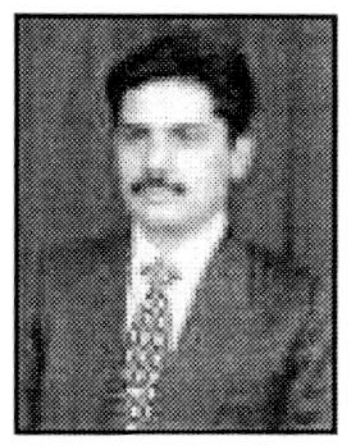

Dr. Rajeev Sharma is an eminent consultant of Homoeopathy, Yoga, Naturopathy and Holistic Medicine in India. He has written more than two hundred books in Hindi and English and around one thousand articles which have been published in various newspapers and magazines. He is also an Editional Board Member of the prestigious *Asian Homoeopathic Journal* besides many other newspapers and magazines.

Dr. Rajeev Sharma has written books on ayurveda, allopathy, homoeopathy, yoga, naturopathy, accupressure, magnetotherapy, reiki, water-therapy, massage and aromatherapy etc.

The books written by Dr. Rajeev Sharma are published by renowned publishers of India. Besides this he is doing editing and translation also. He is content provider to many magazines.

Dr. Rajeev Sharma has written books on all major ailments like diabetes, hypertension, obesity, stomach and respiratiory disorders, E.N.T. disorders, female disorders, UTI disorders, paediatric problems, headache, stress and other mental problems and sexual disorders etc.

Dr. Rajeev Sharma is Medical Advisor to Ralson Remedies (a homoeopathic manufacturer), and Dixit Pharmacy (Ayurvedic Manufacturer), Medical Examiner at the LIC and Medical Officer in U.P. Govt. He has received several prizes for his outstanding achievements. He has been awarded the *Best Author prize in Hindi* by the Ministry of Health and Family Welfare, Government of India and *Sarjana Puraskar by U.P. Hindi Sansthan,* Lucknow. He has delivered talks on All India Radio and lectures on Holistic Medicine in various Government and Non-government Organisations.

He is working as Vastu Fengshui Consultant, Educational Consultant and Marriage and Behaviour Counsellor too.

He is delivering lectures and providing literature on Personality Development and Life Style Management also to the MNC's.

He has established an institute through which you can get certificates by correspondence in Accupressure, Massage, Yoga, Water Therapy, Diet Therapy, Naturopathy, Colour Therapy and Reiki besides other paramedical courses.

Dr. Rajeev Sharma is also a social activist. He has worked a lot against Addition, and prevention of AIDS. Presently he is working to check the population growth of India with an NGO called 'Nav Chetna Manch'. He has worked for pollution control and human rights too and has received the World Human Rights Promotion Award. His name has been published in *LIMCA BOOK OF RECORDS* 2005. He has developed one website too:

www.newkamasutra.com: A site of love, romance and sex.

He is a person of creative mind.He is All India President of an NGO "UTKRISHTA BHARAT" (An All India Association of Socio-Cultural-Religious & Sports Activities).

PREFACE

Homoeopathy is based on symptom similarity. The medicines are selected on the totality of symptoms. This is more than 200 years old science which has benefitted millions of people through out the world. This was originated in Germany by Dr. C. S. F. Hahnemann and was promoted in India in West Bengal first. Guru Ravindra Nath Tagore and Mahatma Gandhi were fond of this science. If symptoms are properly selected and if the medicine is choosen on symptom similarity this science can produce miraculous results.

In this book I have given details of different disorders that too system wise with probable medicines. All the major and common diseases are covered. A chart is given for children's diseases too. There are different chapters on how to take medicines, theory of miasms (disease producing causes), homoeopathic and biochemic medicines details and many more.

If you have any querry you can write to me on sharmarajeev108@rediffmail.com.

CONTENTS

A

HOW TO USE HOMOEOPATHIC MEDICINES ?

Homoeopathic remedies are easy to give and they act rapidly, but they must be used in accordance with the principles of the science discussed here:

The law of similars. Match the symptoms of the patient as closely as possible to the symptoms that were produced in healthy, human beings when the medicine was proved.

The single remedy. Give only one remedy at a time. Each substance is specific to a certain set of disease symptoms; giving two or more remedies at a time introduces unknown elements into the picture: Which medication is causing what effect and how are they interacting?

The minimum dose. This does not refer to the size of the dose but denotes the degree of potentization (6x) in the homeopathically prepared remedy, as explained earlier in this chapter.

The Dosage

The standard dosage in acute ailments is two drops of 30 potency every four hours. To pepare a lotion, simply dissolve one half teaspoon tincture in one cup clean water and apply directly to the affected area.

"Standard dosage" notwithstanding, each case is individual. The interval between doses relates directly to the urgency of the situation, as in an acutely painful condition such as an earache requiring a dose every fifteen minutes. If there is no relief within an hour, you have probably chosen the wrong remedy and need to reassess the case. Homoeopathy requires intelligence, careful observation, and common sense; otherwise, you would be reading the label on a bottle instead of this book!

Continue giving a remedy until improvement starts, then increase the interval between doses; when improvement is well established, discontinue the remedy. Imagine that you are pushing someone on a swing; you give only enough pushes to keep the swing going. Each dose is a push; if you push at the wrong time you may not stop the swinging, but you will interfere with the happy rhythmic motion. Some cases are more clear-cut than others, but if you keep a careful record of the patient's symptoms, you will probably sense when the person is on the mend, or needs another remedy. Prolonged use of a remedy, beyond the time when it is needed, may result in a backlash, or "aggravation"; that is, the patient "proves" the remedy and develops symptoms, as did the test subjects who first took the remedy to find out what it could do.

How to Take a Remedy

To take a remedy, tip the dose onto your clean palm or onto a spoon, and transfer to the tongue. If you are giving the dose to someone else, use his or her palm rather than yours. If you inadvertently pour out more tablets or granules than needed for the dose, discard the excess; do not replace them in the bottle because you may contaminate the remainder of your medicine. When opening the bottle, make certain that nothing touches the inside portion of the cork or cap, and close the bottle as soon as possible. Never have more than one of the remedies open at the same time as contamination can take place through airborne particles.

Medicine should be taken in a clean mouth. By "clean" we mean free of food, drink, tobacco, smoke, toothpaste, mouthwash, mints, or any matter except plain water. It is best not to wash the dose with water: allow it to be absorbed directly through the mucous membrane of the mouth. The best time for taking a remedy is in the morning before breakfast and before brushing the teeth. Put nothing in the mouth except water fifteen minutes before or after the dose.

While taking a homeopathic medicine, avoid any other medicines such as aspirin, laxatives, sleeping pills, and patent medicines of any kind. Do not use nasal drops, antiseptics, liniments, or preparations containing camphor. Saline mouthwash and Calendula antiseptic make good substitutes and will not interfere with homeopathic treatment. Eliminate coffee, which may neutralize the action of the homeopathic remedy.

Storage

Homoeopathic remedies have indefinite shelf life if handled and stored properly. Always keep medicines in the container in which they were supplied; never transfer them to another bottle. This is a good habit to cultivate, as we are dealing with such minute quantities that trace elements of matter, which can cling to the interior of a bottle, may contaminate the fresh supply.

Keep medicines away from strong light, heat, and pungent odors such as camphor, menthol, mothballs, carbolic soap and perfume. As an added protection place your kit in an outer container. If your closet smells of mothballs, a locked bureau drawer is a good storage place. Keep out of reach of small children. A homeopathic remedy, even an entire vial consumed at one gulp, is not toxic or poisonous, but a toddler, intent on sampling the sweet-tasting pills, can wreak havoc on your kit.

B

THE HOMOEOPATHIC HOUSEHOLD KIT

Homoeopathic remedies are supplied in various forms–tablets, granules, and tinctures. Most people prefer the tablet form, in which an alcoholic solution, or dilution, is poured into specially prepared sugar granules that absorb the medication as the alcohol evaporates. Granules are in powder form and are the safest way to administer a remedy if the patient is unconscious. A tincture is an alcoholic solution. Since the concentration of alcohol in a tincture can be irritating, we use the tincture to prepare a lotion as an external remedy to wash and heal the skin. (Another reason for using lotion rather than tincture is to conserve one's supply of tincture.)

The twenty-eight remedies in the kit are in tablet form; each vial, clearly labeled, contains tablets. Vials are stored in a 3½ × 6-inch plastic box with a snap lock.

Inside Your Home Remedy Kit

Homoeopathic remedies are derived from animal; vegetable and mineral sources. Some of these sources, in their crude state, are highly toxic. *Belladonna* is made from a plant, deadly nightshade, that is accurately named; its red berries are poisonous. *Arsenicum alb* is made from the metal arsenic: a deadly poison. The most noxious substances make the most potent healing agents when prepared homoeopathically.

As you may remember from our earlier discussion, the process of preparing homeopathic medicine, potentization (diluting and shaking, or grinding, the substance at each stage of dilution) produces a medicine that contains only trace amounts of the original substance. What is left is the medicinal essence of the substance, or what a physicist has called "energized medicine," so that all homeopathic medicines, regardless of their source, are harmless.

In the following introduction to the twenty-eight most frequently prescribed remedies, I have given the source of each remedy . For a more complete description, see the *Materia Medica* which presents a "personality profile" of each remedy. The symptoms listed are those that provings of the remedy produced in healthy people. When these symptoms match your symptoms, it is probable that particular medicine is YOUR indicated remedy.

Do not expect to digest this information all at once. It is like meeting a roomful of people, in this case, all with foreign names; it takes time to sort them out. Throughout this book, we shall discuss these remedies and many others with their multiple characteristics over and over, so before long their Latin names will no longer sound strange and each will assume a distinct personality. As you gain experience in the use of these remedies, you will undoubtedly come to feel, as a member of a homeopathic study group expressed it, "The remedies are like old friends."

Medicines in the Home Remedy Kit

Aconitum napel/us (monkshood). *Aconite* is useful in the early stages of inflammation of fever and is indicated by the sudden onset of violent symptoms, especially after exposure to dry, cold wind. The patient who needs *Aconite* is fearful, restless, and thirsty for cold drinks.

Allium cepa (red onion). This remedy will help the person with a beginning cold who looks as if he has been peeling onions. There is frequent sneezing and the eyes show a watery discharge and irritation in the nose. The person may also have laryngitis, with a raw sensation extending into the chest.

Antimonium tartaricum (temetic). *Antimonium tart* will benefit the person who has bronchitis and a wheezing cough; mucus in the chest makes a rattling bubbling sound as if the patient were drowning his own secretions. He or she is pale, has a cold sweat and looks sick.

Apis melliflca (honeybee). This remedy will relieve insect bites, including bee stings, or other rosy red spots with stinging pains.

Arnica montana (leopard's bane). Your first thought for the after effects of a fall or overexertion, or injury from a blunt object. The person who needs *Arnica* feels bruised and sore.

Arsenicum album (arsenic). This is the most frequently needed remedy for stomach upsets, vomiting or diarrhea, especially when caused by food poisoning.

Belladonna (deadly nightshade). The *Belladonna* patient is flushed, hot, and restless; symptoms are violent. The person may have a sore throat or cough, headache, earache or fever.

Bryonia alba (white bryonia). *Bryonia* is called the "grumpy bear" because the person who needs it is irritable and wants to be left alone. Whatever the ailment–fever, headache, sore throat, stomach upset–the patient feels worse from the slightest movement and is very thirsty.

Calcarea phosphorica (phosphate of lime). *Calcarea phos* aids in the healing of bones and is therefore prescribed for fractures and difficult teething. This remedy also has a beneficial effect on tonsils and neck glands and on school children's headaches.

Cantharis (Spanish fly). *Cantharis* relieves the frequent, painful urination that occurs in cystitis. It also alleviates the pain of burns and scalds.

Carbo vegetabilis (vegetable charcoal). *Carbo veg* is known as "the great reviver": it helps the person who is on the verge of collapse or whose vitality is low after an illness.

Chamomilla (German chamomile). *Chamomilla* is given to a child when teething is irritable and cranky and just plain impossible. *Chamomilla* is helpful for anyone who is oversensitive to pain, particularly when suffering from a toothache.

Ferrum phosphoricum (phosphate of iron). *Ferrum phos.* helps in the early stages of all inflammatory problems, including head colds, earache, cough, pneumonia, bronchitis, pleurisy and rheumatism.

Gelsemium sempervirens (yellow jasmine). A remedy to consider if the person feels dull, heavy-lidded, complains of aching and chills, is not thirsty and wants to be left alone. *Gelesmium* is often needed for flu, head colds, tension headache.

Hepar sulphuris calcareum (calcium sulphide). *Hepar sulph.* helps to localize inflammation, as in bringing a boil to a head. It is useful for certain types of head colds, sore throat, laryngitis and is the most frequently used remedy for children with croup.

Hypericum perfoliatum (St. John's wort). *Hypericum* heals injured parts rich in nerves, such as fingertips and toes. It also helps tailbone injuries, even old ones.

Ignatia amara (St. Ignatius bean). *Ignatia* is the grief remedy for the person who doesn't recover from an emotional upset such as disappointment or anger; patient sighs very frequently.

Ipecacuanha (ipecac root). *Ipecac* relieves constant nausea with or without vomiting. It also helps to stop a bad nosebleed or bleeding from any part of the body.

Ledum Pal (marsh tea). This is the key remedy for puncture wounds, stings, and bites. *Ledum* is also helpful in eye injuries and in sprained ankle.

Magnesia phosphorica (phosphate of magnesia). Some people call this the "homeopathic aspirin." *Magnesia phos.* eases any spasmodic pain that is relieved by warmth, such as leg cramp, menstrual cramps, or colic.

Mercurius vivus (quicksilver). This remedy is often indicated for tonsillitis, abscessed ears, boils, and gum disease. The person who needs *mercury* is sweaty, feels weak and trembling and is very sensitive to temperature changes.

Nux vomica (poison nut). *Nux* is sometimes called the "hangover remedy" because it often relieves the person who has overindulged in food or alcohol. It also helps the chronic user of laxatives to break the habit.

Phosphorus (phosphorus). Some of the symptoms that indicate a need for *phosphorus* are laryngitis, chest cold, hemorrhage. *Phosphorus* has a long-lasting effect and should not be repeated often.

Pulsatilla (wind flower). This remedy will help a "ripe" cold with profuse thick yellowish discharge. It will also relieve the person who has an upset stomach from eating too much rich food. The person who needs *Pulsatilla* loves the open air, is worse from warmth, is not thirsty,and can't stand fat.

Ruta graveolens (rue). For a shinbone injury or any injury to the periosteum (bone covering). It is also useful for sprains. When

Arnica fails to relieve a bruised, lame feeling resulting from a fall, follow up with *Ruta.*

Spongia tosta (roasted sponge). This remedy's chief symptom is a croupy, wheezing cough, and therefore it is often prescribed for children during an attack of croup.

Sulphur (sublimated sulphur). Homeopaths often prescribe this medication for certain skin diseases that cause dry, itchy skin. *Sulphur* is more often used in chronic diseases than acute ones.

Veratrun album (white hellebore). A remedy for the distressful time when diarrhea and vomiting occur simultaneously. The patient is in a cold sweat, and feels faint. Here is a brief description of the way in which a homeopathic remedy is prepared. Except for the use of machines, the process has not changed since Hahnemann's time.

In preparing *Arnica,* for example, which is extracted from a plant known as leopard's bane, the homeopathic pharmacist dissolves one part of the plant extract, or mother tincture with nine parts of the water /alcohol mixture and vigorously shakes the mixture ten times, striking it with rhythmic sharp downward blows. The result is a 1 x potency. When one part of this first dilution is mixed with nine parts of a fresh alcohol/water solution, again successed ten times, the result is a 2x potency. Continuing this process to the sixth dilution, each time with nine parts of diluent, produces the 6x potency.

If the remedy to be potentized is insoluble in water, as for example, *Mercurius,* the pharmacist grinds the substance to the finest powder, a process called trituration, then mixes one part of this fine powder with nine parts of lactose (milk sugar), and grinds for an hour in a clear mortar to produce the 1 x potency.

Repeating the process with fresh lactose produce the 2x potency; another repetition produce the 3x and so on to the 6x potency we seek.

Higher potencies, because they have proven to be more powerful and deeper acting than lower potencies, should be prescribed only by a physician. The decision as to which potency to prescribe is a complex one and requires many years of study and clinical experience on the part of the homeopathic physician.

You can safely treat your acute ailments with a well-chosen 6x potency, but if you are under the care of a homeopathic physician, you should not treat an acute condition with a remedy without the approval of your doctor.

C

THEORY OF MIASMS

Dr. Hahnemann, the founder of homoeopathy, furthered his concept of miasms by asserting that when there is a chronic case that defies treatment or when even the best selected remedy fails to yield expected results, there is some evidence of hereditary transmittance of the diseases from parents to their offspring and this chain continues unabated unless fully cured.

'Miasm' means pollution or stain which convey the meaning 'Predisposition to chronic disease, whether inherited or developed'. Hence diseases like Syphilis, Psora and Psychosis have a wide-ranging monster. Apart from the recognised three miasms, we can also include AIDS, tuberculosis, certain fevers, cholera, typhoid, diphtheria, gonorrhoea, scabies etc also under 'Miasms'.

In short, combination of two miasms can give birth to a new miasm (for instance AIDS). Allopathy has controlled most of the venereal diseases and cancerous growths, provided the symptoms have been detected at the inital stages when, even a short medicinal course would suffice to affect cure; but late detection of symptoms fails to resolve the crisis when life span may be lengthened for some days/months but such a miserable life is worse than even death.

It is not that all reactive, intractable and incurable cases should always be attributed to 'miasm'. In most of the cases, improper and inadequate selection of a remedy is generally the basic factor. First of all reassess the symptom picture and see where you had faltered or erred. A timely reassessment and revaluation of the case will solve the problem in majority of cases, without even remote reference to Miasmistic theory. It is in chronic cases that one has to look to this theory, when even the best selected remedy fails to show the desired results. In any case, heredity factor must not ever be lost sight of.

In some cases the selected remedy takes a bit longer time to cure, and it is more true in cases where there is lowered phygoctye. Hence a remedy must be afforded a fair time to act, and nothing should be done, say abruptly, by changing the remedy in haste and impatience. In some cases, even fresh symptoms may emerge which must not panic the patient and the doctor.

PSORA

Of all the miasms, Psora is the top ranking miasm to which all the other miasms are secondary. Hahnemann considered Psora as the 'original sin' that caused all other subsequent diseases, as he found it the most destructive, ancient and universal miasm. Psoric miasm is carried by each person and is not possible to eliminate but a correct balance may be established by a suitable anti-psoric remedy. It develops due to a suppressed 'Itch' or 'Scabies.'

Morrison opined that *Psorinum* nosode fully reflected this , miasm, though there are other remedies also but Psorinum leads the list of anti-psoric remedies. Itch, allergies, burning of the skin, congestion or hypersensitivity, hyperactivity are commonly found components of this miasm.

This miasm developed from the suppressed scabies but emanated from the fluid that flowed out of pustules or vesicles which were transmitted by physical contact with the skin–that is, when a healthy person's skin came in contact with an ailing person's skin, the miasm got the 'itch mite', though the infected person may not feel appearance of an eruption of itch for several days after he contracted the miasm from an ailing patient. During this period the 'mite' starts to invade human organism and starts to establish its stronghold. Appearance of eruptions and itching are the forewarning manifestations that psora has made its entry into human body. The actual problem arises when the 'mite' is driven inwardly by the use of certain skin ointments and medicines. Now, at this stage, the 'mite' is driven in and becomes dormant which contribute to triggering of various causes/traumas–by affecting mental, physical and emotional levels. It is a well known conclusion that a suppressed psora affects nervous system which, in turn, adversely affects our hyperactivity and hypersensitivity.

Psora-Related Indications and Symptoms

- Recent or past history of burning sensations and skin disharmony.
- Nervosity, restivity and hurriedness.
- Lack of morals, deceitful, selfish, secretive.
- Lack of courage, timiners, preference of isolation and solitude.
- Inhibitory nature, inability to complete ideas, incohorent articulation/speech.
- Easily tired due to physical debility.
- Low level of self-esteem.
- Mucus membranes generally red and dry.
- Want of or lack of local vital heat.
- Self-reproach and helplessness.

- Any type of discharge makes him feel better.
- Worse while standing.
- Bruised, sore feeling, especially when pains are of neuralgic origin/type.
- A "burnt taste in the mouth".
- Poor memory or forgetfulness.
- Constipation.
- Hypertension, hypersensitivity, hyperactivity, hypothyrodism.
- Tendency to save/hoard many things.
- Fear of being totally alone or any failure continues to haunt him.
- Overweight.
- Poor and slow metabolism.
- Reappearance of skin disharmony improves many symptoms.
- Averse to milk, but pines and desires for spicy, fried, saltish and sweetish foods.
- Activity, warmth, all discharges, summer and heat conditions, lying down make him better but he feels worse in winter, cold, on/while standing and during sleep.
- Almost all the illnesses, arising out of or due to Psora, manifest themselves around 40th year of age.

Specific Anti-Psoric Remedies, with leading symptoms

APIS : Itching, burning and stinging sensations.

ARSENIC IOD : It is a warm-blooded Arsenic Album.

ARESNIC ALBUM: Restivity and burning sensations.

HEPAR SULPH : Irritability and hypersensitivity.

LACHESIS: When discharges ensue, improvement ushers in.

LYCOPODIUM: Sensitive, weak, selfish, timid and insecure.

NATRUM MUR : Weakness for salty food. Allergies, prefers solitude.

NITRIC ACID: Anxious, irritable, hypersensitive, negative.

PSORINUM (PRINCIPAL REMEDY) : Hopeless, anxious, chilly, conscious of poverty, filthy and dirty.

SELENIUM: Skin disharmony, despair, irritable and theorising.

SEPIA: Preeminently a woman's remedy. Irritable low esteem, fatigued, sits cross legs lest private parts escape out of vagina; constipation.

SULPHUR: Burning sensations, aversion to bathing; worse standing. It unmasks dormant symptoms.

ZINCUM MET: Complaining nature, oversensitive, restless and irritable.

TRY ALSO: *Aloe, Calcarea, Phos, Clematis, Silicea, Mezerium, Graphites, Stannum,* Petroleum, Sarsaparilla.

"Lack" and "overall insufficiency" explain many traits of Psora that affect all spheres; puts a damper on well-being, recovery, growth, motivation, career opportunities. Such limiting factors extend to and engulf episodes of apathy, fear, indifference, depression, anxiety, ability. No doubt a psoric person is full of ideas but is unable to translate his plans into action due to emotional, mental or physical constraints and compulsions. It is the performance that gets affected.

Sense of worthlessness, inability to express mental reservations to others, force the patients to seek solitude. They feel that by keeping aloof, they can be more safe and secure. Psoric manifestations percolate to sycosis and appearance of tumors and warts is an indication of the psora miasm intruding into the sycotic miasm.

SYCOSIS

Past history of a "Fig Wart" disease is considered to be causative factor of sycotic miasm which develops due to "suppressed gonorrhoea". When the growths were surgically removed or burnt off, the disease seemed to have been eliminated but, in fact, the disease developed internally that created a secondary disharmony which appeared after many years.

Top ranking anti-sycotic remedy namely *Medorriunum,* was introduced by Dr. Burnett who is a pioneer figure in introducing Nosodes in homeopathic system. Small Pox Vaccine was considered an analogous remedy to Medor. But the former had many a damaging side effect, hence it didn't find favour with the physicians. The nosode is prepared from (an untreated) discharge of gonorrhoea that contains the bacteria and the human tissue but its toxic virulence is removed by potentization method of homoeopathy.

Typical Symptoms of Sycotic Miasm

- Vertigo and Dizziness.
- Hyperactive, restless, cruel, suspicious.
- Perforation of tissues, growths and tumors.
- Fails to recollect/memorise recent events.
- Selfish, deceitful, quarrelsome, humiliation.

- Low esteem, condemnation or self-reproachment/self-denunciation.
- Fits of rage/anger, thoughts of destruction or else suicidal tendencies.
- Loses threads/chain of thoughts/conversation or forgets words.
- Tendency to irritating teasing coughs bronchitis and asthma.
- Gout and joint pains, leucorrhoea, menstural pains, inflammatory pelvic disease.
- Moles, loss of smell, hay fever, chronic nasal discharge(s).
- Growth of warts improves mental conditions.
- Thermic changes worsen symptoms.
- Enlargment of prostate (Prostatitis), appendicitis, ringworms.
- Fishy odour/taste and excessive perspiration.
- Aversion to wine, spices and milk, but desires meat, fatty food, salt, beers, seasoned foods, peppers.
- Amelioration from movement, dry weather, winter and atmosphere.
- Growths, tumors, cysts, jaundice, liver spots, freckles. Aggravations from heat, damp, cold and rainy seasons, humidity.

Remedies Closely Related to Syotic Miasm

ARGEN MET: Vertigo, sudden appearance of pains.

KALI IOD : Asthma, hay fever, arthritis, cruel and irritable.

KALI SULPH : Asthma, headaches, low confidence and irritability.

LYCOPODIUM: Herpes, leucorrhoea, perspiration, low esteem.

MEDORRHINUM : Chronic discharges, herpes.

NAT. SULPH : Warts, mental dullness, gonorrhoea, suicidal tendency.

NITRIC ACID: Vaginitis, negative and irritable, herpes, cursting.

RADIUM BROMIDE: Tickling cough, joint's affections and gout; mole, irritability.

SEPIA: Fishy odour, herpes, PMS, irritability, mental dullness.

TARENTULA: Hyper restivity, tumors, deceitful and destructive.

THUJA : Gonorrhoea, warts, herpes, feeling of worthlessness, secretive.

STAPHYSAGRIA : Anger, low esteem, shame, self reproach, low confidence.

OTHER REMEDIES: Ars, Alb, Ars Iod, Mezereum, Nat Mur, Psorinum, Pyrogen, Lachesis, Sarsparilla and Silicea.

Due to malfunctioning of pituitary gland, cretinism/dwarfism surface. There is also lack of coordination that results in body's incompetence to absorb and assimilate energy. Disharmony of sexual organs surfaces in the form of multiple sexual upsets. Medorrhinum has been described as the sex, drugs, rock and roll remedy when excess is involved, though Thuja is another striking remedy which can cure 'Fig Warts' and such other manifestations.

No medicine should be administered merely on the basis of a solitary symptom but all the leading indications must also be taken into account. Moreover, causes of other symptoms should also be tackled alongside the leading symptom and concomitant symptoms, for the simple reason that we are treating a patient holistically and not in isolation.

SYPHILIS

This is the last and third chronic miasm that stems from suppression of syphilis (another venereal disease) and results from a sexual intercourse. To say that syphilis is caused by illicit contact (sexual) with a prostitute is simply a denial of truth, as any woman can suffer from this infection and pass on the infection to man, and then again from man to woman and so on and so forth. First it is a pustule, then a discharge that appears after 24 weeks after exposure. If controlled at the inception stage, it can be cured but, in chronic stage, it is liable to adversely affect other organs. A pregnant syphilitic lady may pass on the infection to her developing foetus. There is hardly any organ in the body which can remain unaffected by this infection. But, once the malady, with all its attendant symptoms, has been fully cured, on the basis of negative findings, it is not going to reccur unless one gets again infected. Once fully treated, it can neither be transmitted to the mating partner nor to the off-spring.

Typical Symptoms of Syphilitic Miasm

- Forgetful, mental dullness, sadness and depression.
- Longing for solitude, predisposition to suicide, desire to kill.
- Highly secretive even about his own pains.
- Wickedness, perversion, pessimist with fixed and rigid ideas.
- Hair greasy and oily, with large head and ears.

- Loss of smell, metallic taste in the mouth.
- Asymmetrical teeth
- Oldish appearance and wrinkled face.
- Thin and spoon-shaped nails.
- Low sexual desires (in rare cases highly sexual urge).
- Pains in almost all the bones and ulcers on skin.
- Aversion for animal foods and meat.
- Longings for sour, indigestible things, cold foods, stimulants and smoking.
- Worse summer, warmth, at seashore, night and by night sweats.
- Better: Temperate climate, cold, sunshine, change of position.

Highly Suitable Anti-syphilitic Remedies

AURUM MET : Aversion to meet, suicidal tendency, depressed, pains worse at night time.

FLUORIC ACID : Indifferent materialistic outlook, isolated, weak nails.

HEPAR SULPH : Skin ulcers, offensive odours, suicide, sensitive and irritable.

KALI IOD : Worse at night, harsh tempered and cruel.

KALI SULPH : Bone pains, warm blooded, depressed and low esteem.

LACHESIS : Introvert, jealous, suspicious, hot.

MECRC SOL : Profuse and high perspiration, low confidence, sensitive.

NITRIC ACID : Cursing, angry, selfish, fearful, hypersesitive, chilly.

PHYTOLACCA : Sore throat, mastitis; general soreness, restivity, shamelessness.

SILICEA : Sensivitve and yielding, lacks stamina, low esteem, constipation.

SYPHILINUM : Destructive, compulsive, pains and chilliness, dread of night.

NOTE : **Syphilinum** is the leading remedy, followed closely by Silica, Hepar sulph, Merc. Sol, and Nitric Acid.

TRY ALSO : Arsenic Alb, Calc. Ars, Conium, Iodatum, Lyco, Ledum, Phos, Phos. acid, Staphysagria.

Pre-dispostion/suppression generally surface around the 40th year either on mental, physical or emotional levels. The patient is bound to suffer from host of skin manifestations like psoriasis, eczema, ulcers, pus or blood filled discharges (which are quite offensive), gangrene and rare itching. Whenever you find symptoms like sterility, cancer, abortions, heart problems, tuberculosis, suicide, blindness, insanity etc, you can easily trace back to family history of syphilitic miasm which, if untreated and fully eliminated (rather rooted out), will pass on from one generation to another. The syphilitic patient is so secretive and self-confined that he won't let out his reactions and emotions. His inner feeling of worthlessness makes him deceitful and dishonest. These persons have no sympathy for others but would expect others to feel sorry for them and show sympathy.

Finally, get yourself fully checked up at the inception stage or when you notice any of the above symptoms(s). A timely cure will not only save the sufferer but also the wife or husband and the off-spring.

TUBERCULAR MIASM

Low grade fever, persistent and exhausting cough or cough bouts, lowered vitality, gradual weight loss, dry skin, cough with blood-spitting, pain in cesht, lungs and throat, cold perspiration, cyanotic skin, exhausting, wasting away of general strength are some of the symptoms which might be regarded as forewarning signals pointing to presence of tuberculosis which is a steady and gradually progressing disease and, if untreated, may pass on to all those who come into contact with the patient. It is a hereditary disease and when history of family is taken it is found (though not always) that some member from the maternal and or paternal side had suffered from this wasting disease.

Tuberculosis may engulf intestines, bones, muscles, tissues, skin, lungs or may affect any other organs also. Though symptoms and etiological factors do vary in each variety, the most common factor remains the same. There is hardly any miasmatic literature available on tubercular miasm and the symptoms have been detailed only under tuberculosis and it is equally true of cancer miasm. Except for the mental symptoms, which primarily are related to this miasm, all other symptoms have been detailed under 'Tuberculosis'.

General Symptoms (not miasmatic symptoms)

- Tendency to catch cold at the slightest exposure.
- Overall weakness and general wasting away of vital force and resistance.
- Frightful dreams and insomnia.

- Desire for open air, change of place and climate. Worse in winter, cold winds and rainy seasons.
- Irritability, agitated temper and depression.
- Aversion to mental work and physical activity and breathless, longing for fresh air (due to lack of oxygen).

Symptoms of Tubercular Miasm

- Worse from greasy and oily foods, at night, during thunderstorms but better in open and dry air, day time.
- Aversion for fat or meat.
- Longings and penchant for potatoes, greasy objects, tobacco, fats, salts, indigestible things.
- Intolerant and dissatisfied with everything.
- Frequent change of jobs, places and relationships.
- Quick changes in attitudes, moods.
- Indifference and depression, but no hopelessness.
- Careless, irritable, angry, quarrelsome.
- Inability to concentrate and uncontrollable passions.
- Fear of dogs. Weakness with fatigue.
- Periodic headaches, glandular affections.
- Natural discharges often improve the condition.
- Easy flushing of face with circumscribed spots.
- Offensive odours, hay fever and allergies.
- Freckles, eczema, impetigo, herpes, ulcers in mouth, cheasy ear discharges.
- Uncontrollable passions.
- Hypersensitive to weather changes.

Leading Remedies for Tubercular Miasm

ARS. IOD : Restivity, glandular infections, asthma, allergies, depressed spirits, eczema.

BACILLINUM : Easily cathes to cold, depressed, irritable, humid asthma.

BARYTA CARB : Glands wasting away, mouth ulcers, feels better in open air.

CALC. CARB : General weakness, multiple allergies, fear of dogs, despaired of recovery.

HEPAR SULPH : Chilly, glandular swellings, irritability, anxiety, hypersensitivity.

IODUM : Changeable and hurried mood, fatigue and debility, wasting away, asthma, hay fever.

TUBERCULINUM : Allergies, tuberculosis, asthma, loves travelling.

TRY ALSO: Calc.Phos, Lyco, Natrum, Zincum Met, All Kali salts, Hydrastis, Puls, Spongia, Sulphur, Tarantula, Nitric Acid, Carcinocin, Carbo Animalis, Sanicula.

Tubercular miasm also fits in "problem children" showing symptoms, like throwing away things, striking, biting, head banging, screaming, attention deficit orders, malicious and destructive.

As for adults, they have tendency to grow more thinned and emaciated but desire travel which they are unable to undertake. Their mental alertness is not consistent with their fatigue and physical emaciation.

Other Symptoms of Tubercular Diathesis

- Family history of allergies and tuberculosis, worms and/ or ringworms.
- "Pigeon. chest" or a "caved in" chest.
- Hair dry and thin.
- Bleeding from rectum or nose.
- Nails have white spots, break and split away quite easily, are stained or wavy.

In any case, remedies like Tuberculmum must not be repeated frequently nor given in higher doses, as it can imperil life itself. Concentrate on avoiding overstimulations and aggravating factors. So called "new strains" are simply a convequence of the older ones, hence the physician shouldn't feel concerned nor scare the patient. It is pointed out that tuberculosis, of any etiology, is fully manageable and curable, even at a later stage but then, freedom from disease or relapse cannot be guaranteed. The patient has to take all the advised precautions. The physician can only advise but only the patient knows in which season and by ingestion of which food items aggravate his symptoms. You can only motivate, guide and induce but cannot force the patient. Precaution and abstinence are the two watchwords which tubercular patients must not lose sight of.

CANCER

Any 'growth' must not be mistaken for a cancerous growth. Cancerous tumors (growths) can be subdivided into following categories, viz.

(*i*) **Carcinoma:** It is a malignant growth of epithelial, cells, and

(*ii*) **Sarcoma:** Its malignancy develops from connective tissue of muscle, bone or tendons.

Human body is endowed with an immune system which, in fact, is body's defence mechanism but it is also inundated with germs and bacteria of various types. Most of the infections are controlled by our immune system that forces out the invading intruders. When body's immune and defence mechanism is weak in factors, like stress, lack of physical activity, pollutions and toxicants, malnutritioned diet, poor hygiene, climatic changes, further render the body weak and susceptible to infections. Some of the mentioned factors are well within our control but other depend on factors beyond our control, and pre-disposition to cancerous growth tops the list of infection.

Since cancer is still an unresolved and baffling disorder for the medical community, I would dwell upon certain factors that are held, or at least said, to cause cancerous growth.

Warning Signals

- Persistent pain occuring at one organ.
- Bleeding from any orifice (opening) of the body, including skin.
- Appearance of tumorous growth, whether benign or malignant, in or around any organ.
- Cancer may affect any part of the body but more particularly, brain, throat, mouth, oesophagus, liver, stomach, intestines, nose, rectum, anus or any bone, tissue or even skin, breasts, vagina, uterus, prostrate, kidneys etc.

Symptomatic indications

- Pains having no apparent cause.
- Chronic hoarasness and undue strain on vocal cords.

- Exhaustion, fatigue and general run-down condition.
- Malignant growths, moles, warts, protrusions.
- Continuous low grade fever.
- Constant urge to clear the throat, feels as if something is lodged therein.
- Fears and anxieties rise without any discernible cause.
- Digestive problems, chronic constipation, bleeding, pain, tensesmus.
- Patient is better with family members and friends and feels worse when alone.
- Needs nurturing, support.
- Feels worse at night, especially when alone.
- Ulcerations in mouth, skin.
- Unusual lumps and hardness.

In cancer, even well chosen and selected remedies fail to act, as in the case of other miasmistic disorders, hence one may have to resort to 'Method of error and trial' but not of 'Hit and run'.

Suggested Remedies

1. Hydrastis
2. Lachesis
3. Arrenic Alb
4. Calcarea Ars
5. Carbo Animals
6. Nitric Acid
7. Phytolacca
8. Carcinosin

Try also: Bromium, Chelidonium, Iodum, Kreosote, Phosphorus, Alumina, Calc.Carb, Cadm Sulph, Bufo, China, Graphites, CarboVeg, KaliArs, Merc.Sol, Ignatia, Natrum Carb, Natrum Mur, Thuja, Sulphur, Zincum, Kali cyan, Silicea, Echinacea, Cistus, Condur, Conium, Galium Acid, Kreosote, Symphytum.

Specific Remedies

Cancer of Antrum - Aurum, Symphytum.

Bone Cancer - Aur. Iod, Phos, Symphytum.

Cancer of breast - Ars lod, Bar. lod, Brom, Bufo, *Carbo Anim,* Carcinocin, Candur, *Conium,* Acid Formic, Graph, *Hydrastis,* Phyto, *Plumb lad,* Scirrhin.

Cancer of lower bowel - Bufo

Cancer of Caecum - Ornithog

Cancer of Glandular Structures - Hoang Nan, Cancer of Uterus - *Aur.Mur.Nat,* Carbo An, Carcin, Fuligo, Hydras, lod, Lapis Alb, NitAcid.

Cancer of Stomach - Acetic Acid, *Ars.Alb,* Bism, Cad. Sulph, *Condur,* Acid Formic, *Hydras,* Kreos, Phos, Secale cor.

Remedies to Relieve Pain of Cancer

Apis, Anthrac, *Arsenic Alb,* Aster, Bry, *Calc. Ac,* Calc. Carb, Calc. Ox, Carcinos, Cedran, Cinnamon, Condur, Con, Echin, *Euphorb, Hydras,* Mag Phos, Morph, Opium, Ovat, Phos Ac, Silicea.

Note: If cancerous growth is spreading its tantacles to adjoining tissues and also doesn't yield to any type of oral/local treatment, surgical one should undertake surgical treatment without delay.

Cancer of lower bowel - Bufo

Cancer of Caecum - Ornithog

Cancer of Glandular Structures - Hoang Nan, Iod. Cancer of Uterus - *Aur.Mur.Nat,* Carbo An, Carcin, Fuligo, Hydras, lod, Lapis Alb, NitAcid.

Cancer of Stomach - Acetic Acid, *Ars.Alb,* Bism, Cad. Sulph, *Condur,* Acid Fornic, *Hydras,* Kreos, ornithog, Phos, Secale cor.

Remedies to Relieve Pain of Cancer

Apis, Anthrac, *Arsenic Alb,* Aster, Bry, *Calc. Ac,* Calc. Carb, Calc. Ox, Carcinos, Cedran, Cinnamon, Condur, Con, Echin, *Euphorb, Hydras,* Mag Phos, Morph, Opium, Ovat, Phos Ac, Silicea.

1

TEETH AND DIGESTIVE DISORDERS

Teeth Disorders

Teething

Some children have no problems at all when their first teeth break through. For others, it is quite an ordeal, and for their parents as well.

Symptoms

The most common symptoms of teething are pain in the teeth and gums, drooling, redness and swelling of the gums, fever, changes in the stool, restlessness, fussiness, and difficult sleeping.

Complications

Teething can be a challenging event, even though there are no complications.

Finding the Homeopathic Medicine

- If the baby is chubby, contented, sweaty on the back of his head, and slow to teethe, give Calcarea carbonica.
- For babies who are beside themselves and inconsolable when they teethe and whose tantrums are outrageous, give Chamomilla.
- If she is peevish and nothing pleases her, but not as fussy as described for Chamomilla, give Calcarea phosphorica.
- If Calcarea phosphorica doesn't work, give Chamomilla.

- If the baby has delicate features, is constipated, and is slow to teethe, give Silica.

Self Care and Home Remedies

- Giving the baby something cold to chew on often relieves discomfort. This can be a pacifier or teething ring that has been put briefly in the freezer, or ice wrapped in a clean, wet cloth.
- If you cannot find homeopathic medicines, give the baby dilute chamomile tea.
- If you cannot find any single homeopathic medicines and you are desperate, try the homeopathic combination teething tablets. (Biocombination No. 21)

Toothache

Pain in the teeth, sometimes involving the gums and mucous membranes.

Symptoms

The pain may range from mild to severe, and is often affected by chewing, hot and cold, and draft. Common causes of tooth pain are tooth decay, dental abscesses, nerve sensitivity, dental work, sinus infections, trauma, and damage to the facial nerve.

Complications

Complications include abscesses, death of a nerve (necessitating a root canal), loss of a tooth, or a severe, untreated infection that can become systemic.

Finding the Homeopathic Medicine

- For severe dental pain with irritability, give Chamomilla or Hepar sulphuris.

- If drinking coffee aggravates the pain, give Chamomila.
- For toothaches relieved by slashing cold water in the mouth, give Coffea.
- If the pain is due to a sensitive dental abscess, give Hepar sulphuris.
- If the toothache is accompanied by bad breath, a coated tongue, and a lot of salivation, give Mercurius.
- If the toothache is unbearable and is limited to the left side of the face, consider Plantago.

Self Care and Home Remedies

- Ice may temporarily numb the pain.
- Clove oil acts as an analgesic, but may interfere with homeopathic medicines.
- Take white willow bark or another pain reliever temporarily until the homeopathic medicines have a chance to act.

Digestive Disorders

Amebic Dysentery

Amebiasis is a parasitic infection caused by a microganism called Entamoeba bistolytica, more commonly known as amebas. It is usually contracted by ingesting cysts in drinking water or food contaminated with stool. It is more frequent in parts of the world where sanitation is poor, and is a problem often encountered by travelers to developing countries.

Symptoms

The main symptoms of amebic dysentery are painful abdominal cramps, loose watery stools, and gas. The stools may contain mucus and blood, and are infectious. Amoebas frequently cause liver swelling and tenderness and, less commonly, abscesses in the liver. The diagnosis is confirmed primarily by a laboratory examination of the stool called an "ova and parasite" test. Sometimes several stool samples are needed to find the amebas.

Complications

Since amoebias is may be confused with ulcerative colitis, irritable bowel syndrome, and other parasitic infections, diagnosis by a qualified medical professional is recommended. Dehydration, blood loss, and death are posible complications.

Finding the Homeopathic Medicine

- If the person is extremely anxious and restless with diarrhea, give Arsenicum album.
- If the person has exhausting diarrhoea with cramps, give Arsenicum album and Podophyllum.
- If the stool is explosive, consider Croton tiglium, Gambogia, or Podophyllum.
- If there is significant nausea and vomiting, first consider Ipecac, then Arsenicum album.
- If there is lots of rumbling and gurgling in the abdomen, give Podophyllum, Croton tiglium, or Gambogia.
- If there is profuse diarrhea and cramping with sweating and shivering, first think of Veratrum album then Arsenicum album.

Self Care and Home Remedies

- Drink plenty of fluids and replenish electrolytes, including sodium and potassium. Electrolyte solutions available from pharmacies are useful.

- Clear liquids such as water, vegetable broth, and diluted fruit juice help replace fluids.
- The diet should be light and bland; include vegetable soup, whole-grain toast, brown rice, bananas, and apple sauce.
- A warm pack over the abdomen is soothing and may reduce cramping.
- One tablespoon of psyllium seed husks per day often helps to firm up stools.

Colic

Colic is a condition found in babies from just after birth until three or four months of age, with crying, irritability, and what seems to be pain or cramps in the abdomen. They usually seem quite hungry, eat and gain weight normally, and particularly like to suck. The actual cause and process by which colic happens are unknown.

Symptoms

Colicky babies cry and appear to be in pain or distress. Gas may be part of the problem. They may cry incessantly, or only at certain times. The crying can be very distressing to parents, who feel helpless to do anything aboutit.

Complications

Simple colic is not life-threatening, not does it lead to any serious illness. It usually passes on its own in a matter of weeks. If the baby doesn't gain weight, vomits excessively, or has persistent diarrhea, medical attention should be sought to determine the cause of the problem.

Finding the Homeopathic Medicine

- If the baby can't seem to tolerate milk, first think of Aethusa, then Magnesia phosphorica, Calcarea carbonica or Lycopodium.
- If there is a tendency toward frequent belching, and the baby seems to feel better after belching, Carbo vegetabilis is needed.
- For colic in extremely fussy, irritable babies, especially if they arch their backs and areinconsolable, consider Chamomilla.
- If a baby doubles over with the colic or brings his knees up to his chest, think of Colocynthis first then Magnesia phosphorica.
- For colic with excessive bloating and gas, particularly if the baby seems to be worse after ingesting milk, look at Magnesia phosphorica.

Self Care and Home Remedies

- Make sure the baby has been burped after eating.
- Rocking, carrying or holding the baby may soothe him.
- Gripe water is available in many grocery stores.
- Pacifiers may help with the uge to suck.
- Swaddling the baby fairly tightly and placing her on her stomach may help.
- A hot water bottle placed on the baby's abdomen may relieve discomfort.

Constipation

Constipation means difficulty in passing stool, or the inability to have a bowel movement when desired. It can be caused by diseases affecting the bowel or nervous system, emotional stress, lack of bowel tone and peristalsis, insufficient fiber in the diet, dehydration, lack of exercise, drugs and, rarely, obstruction of the bowel.

Symptoms

Hard, dry, or soft stool, pain on having a bowel movement, gas and bloating and hemorrhoids are the main symptoms. Feelings of sluggishness, mental dullness, bad breath and body odour often accompany constipation.

Complications

Acute constipation mainly causes discomfort. If it persists, impaction of the hard, dry stool can occur, blocking the rectum and requiring manual removal. Enlargement of segments of the colon may occur if constipation is chronic and severe.

Finding the Homeopathic Medicine

For constipation that is due to dryness with no urge, in a person who seems confused, consider Alumina.

- A person who needs Bryonia has large, hard stools with dryness, and a lot of thirst for cold drinks; many symptoms are worse from motion.
- For a stubborn, chilly flabby person who sweats on his head and has stubborn constipation, try Calcarea carbonica.
- When there is dryness, and a dreamy, drowsy, dizzy state, give Nux moschata.
- When the person is an irritable businessperson, consider Nux vomica or Bryonia.
- If the person has constant urges but can't go, even with a lot of straining, try Nux vomica.

- For constipation during pregnancy and menstruation, and a feeling like a ball in the anus or that the rectum and uterus will fall out, consider Sepia.
- For bashful stool (comes out part way, then recedes) in a refined, shy person with sweaty feet, try Silica.

Self Care and Home Remedies

- Drink eight glasses of water per day, starting with a glass of warm water with lemon immediately on rising in the morning.
- Eat lots of fresh fruits and vegetables, at least half of them raw.
- Eat whole grains and supplement with a tablespoon of bran stirred in juice or baked in muffins or in cereal.
- Take a one to three km. walk daily.

Diarrhea

Acute diarrhea is usually due to infection by such bacteria as Staphylococcus, E. coli, Salmonella, or Shigella or such parasites as Amebas or Giardia lamblia. Infection may come from eating or drinking contaminated food or water. Some diarrhea is caused by emotional or digestive upset.

Symptoms

The stools are loose or watery, sometimes profuse or explosive and foul-smelling. Food particles may be found in the stool.

Complications

Diarrhea often results in loss of fluids and electrolytes such as sodium and potassium, which must be replaced to prevent dangerous levels of dehydration and electrolyte imbalance. Homeopathic medicines can stop diarrhea, but rehydration is still important.

Finding the Homeopathic Medicine

If stool is like jelly due to mucus, give Aloe.

- If the person is chilly, anxious, nervous and restless, Arsenicum album is your best bet.
- If diarrhea comes immediately after eating or drinking, look at Croton tiglium and Gambogia.
- If there is a lot of rectal itching with the diarrhea, combined with urgency first thing in the morning, Sulphur is indicated.
- If the diarrhea is violent and is accompanied by profuse sweating and chills, give Veratrum album.

Self Care and Home Remedies

Drink plenty of fluids and replenish such electrolytes as sodium and potassium. Electrolyte solutions available from pharmacies are useful. Clear liquids such as water, vegetable broth and diluted fruit juice help replace fluids.

The diet should be light and bland, including vegetable soup, whole grain toast, brown rice, bananas, and applesauce.

A warm pack over the abdomen is soothing and may reduce cramping. Calcium and Magnesium (500 mg per day) may also help to reduce cramping.

One tablespoon psyllium seed husks per day often helps to firm up stools.

Gas

Gas is a byproduct of fermentation or rotting of food in the digestive tract by yeast and bacteria. It may be odorless or foul smelling. Fermentation produces carbon dioxide, which has no smell. Bacteria often produce methane and hydrogen sulfide, which do have a foul smell.

Symptoms

Belching, passing gas and abdominal bloating with rumbling sounds are the most common symptoms of gas.

Complications

Gas may be painful if it is trapped in the stomach or intestines. More serious abdominal problems are sometimes mistaken for simple gas pains. If gas doesn't resolve within six to twelve hours, or is very severe or accompanied by fever, nausea, and vomiting, seek medical attention to get a proper diagnosis of the abdominal pain.

Finding the Homeopathic Medicine

- If bloating is extreme or if the person is exhausted or collapsed and wants to be fanned, give Carbo vegetabilis.
- If the person is doubled over in pain and doubling over makes him feel better, give Colocynthis.
- When gas and bloating take away the appetite, and the person lacks confidence and is worse from 4:00 to 8:00 pm., give Lycopodium.
- If the person is chilly, irritable and impatient and can't seem to pass the gas without straining, give Nux vomica.
- When the person is weepy, changeable and clingy and has eaten too much fat or rich food, give her Pulsatilla.

Self Care and Home Remedies

- Charcoal capsules are helpful in relieving gas. Take two capsules every four hours.
- Lying on the back and bringing the knees to the chest may cause gas to pass.
- Squatting helps relieve gas.
- Massaging the abdomen in a clockwise direction helps the lower bowel gas to pass.
- Babies may be burped over the shoulder.
- Treat constipation to relieve chronic gas.

Eliminate gas forming foods from the diet, such as beans, potatoes, sweets, and carbonated drinks.

Hemorrhoids

Hemorrhoids are varicose veins of the rectum. They may be inside the rectum, or they may protrude outward through the anus. They most commonly result from constipation or pregnancy, and may also be associated with liver problems.

Symptoms

The most annoying symptom associated with hemorrhoids is pain due to inflammation and swelling. This may range from a mild discomfort with or without itching, to pain so severe that sitting or having a bowel movement is excruciating. Hemorrhoids often bleed.

Complications

Blood clots may become lodged in the hemorrhoidal veins surrounding the hemorrhoid. The hemorrhoids may ulcerate and bleed profusely. Other possible causes of rectal bleeding should be investigated, including colitis, polyps and tumors.

Finding the Homeopathic Medicine

- If the main symptom is pain like small sharp sticks in the rectum, consider Aesculus and Collinsonia.
- If swelling and bleeding are prominent, think first of Hamamelis.
- If the person is chilly, over stressed, and drinks too much alcohol, consider Nux vomica.
- In a warm blooded person with lots of the rectal itching and recal spasms, give Sulphur.

Self Care and Home Remedies

- Take a sitz bath. Fill the bathtub with hot water to two inches below the navel. sit with knees bent. Stay in the tub for five minutes. Then squat in a tub of cold water for one minute. Repeat the cycle to three times.
- Take 1000 milligrams of bioflavonoids daily to strengthen the capillaries.
- Keep the rectal area clean.
- If you are constipated, drink plenty of water and take one tablespoon of bran, flaxseed oil, or psyllium seed one to two times daily until the constipation is relieved.
- Avoid spicy foods, they may aggravate the hemorrhoids.
- Get exercise to increase circulation in the pelvic area.
- Peel a garlic clove, scratch its surface several times and insert in the rectum as a suppository. Remove after eight hours or when the stool is passed.

Heaptitis

Hepatitis is an inflammation of the liver, usually of viral origin, but it may also be caused by drugs or alcoholism. Hepatitis A is transmitted by contact with contaminated water or food, stool, blood, or secretions. Hepatitis B is transmitted primarily through blood transfusions or contaminated needles. Hepatitis C occurs mostly after blood transfusions, causing acute hepatitis that may become chronic. Legally it is necessary to call the local health department to report a newly diagnosed case of hepatitis.

Symptoms

Overall weakness or discomfort, nausea and vomiting, diarrhea, poor appetite, and fever are the main symptoms. Jaundice may be marked, depending on the stage of the hepatitis. Hives and joint pains may also occur.

Complications

Hepatitis causes severe liver dysfunction with jaundice, bloating, and diarrhea, and may be fatal in extreme cases. Hepatitis may become chronic, causing long term liver damage that can be fatal.

Finding the Homeopathic Medicine

- The most common medicines are Chelidonium, china and Lycopodium.
- If there is considerable right shoulder blade pain, give Chelidonium.
- If the person has a history of gonorrhea or chlamydia, he probably needs Natrum sulphuricum.
- If perspiration and the breath smell bad and there is excessive saliva, give mercurius.
- If the person has a strong craving for cold drinks, look at Phosphorus.

Self Care and Home Remedies

- Get a hepatitis screen to determine the type of hepatitis you have.

- Make sure that the local public health department has been contacted.
- Eat a light, low-fat diet with lots of fruits and vegetables, especially beets.
- Take Vitamin C, 1000 mg three times a day.
- Take liver herbs, including danelion root, milk thistle, or beet greens.

Indigestion and Heartburn

Indigestion and heartburn are common conditions following eating too much or not being able to digest food properly.

Symptoms

Indigestion can include nausea, gas, belching, stomach pain, and heart burn. It usually occurs in the two hours immediately after eating. Heart burn is burning pain in the chest behind the sternum, which is associated with the reflux of acidic or caustic stomach fluids into the esophagus. Heartburn may occur after eating any food which stimulates acid production in the stomach, such as proteins, spicy foods, or chocolate.

Complications

Indigestion and heartburn are usually uncomplicated, and respond easily to change in diet, antacids, or homeopathic treatment. The symptoms may be confused with symptoms of a stomach ulcer, a hiatal hernia, or angina. If indigestion is severe or persistent, medical attention should be sought to determine the cause of the problem.

Finding the Homeopathic Medicine

- When extreme burnig pain is the main symptom, along with a lot of anxiety and restlessness, think of Arsenicum, especially in a self centered person who wants support and has many fears.

- Lycopodium is the medicine if the person is insecure yet bossy and full of false bravado, gets lots of gas from just a little food, and is worse from 4:00 to 8:00 P.M.
- When the person is irritable, impatient and hard-driving, and suffers from too much rich food, coffee and alcohol, give Nux vomica.
- Conversely, when the person suffers from rich food, but is mild, gentle, changeable and weepy and wants to be taken care of, think of Pulsatilla.
- If the person is lazy, intellectual, egotistical and sloppy and suffers from heartburn and morning diarrhea, give Sulphur.

Self Care and Home Remedies

- Avoid overeating, especially heavy or rich foods.
- Avoid fats, spicy foods, alcohol, coffee, and chocolate.
- Commercial antacids may provide temporary relief.
- Charcoal capsules are helpful in relieving gas. Take two capsules every four hours.
- Lying on the back and bringing the knees to the chest may cause gas to pass.
- Squatting helps gas to pass.
- Eliminate gas producing foods from the diet, such as beans, potatoes, sweets, and carbonated drinks.

Nausea and Vomiting

Nausea and vomiting are symptoms of digestive distress that can come from many causes, including strong odors, morning sickness, motion sickness, food poisoning, indigestion, intestinal obstruction, alcohol intoxication, drug use, prescription drugs, chemotherapy, and exposure to toxic materials, as well as emotional causes such as anxiety, stage fright, and disgust.

Symptoms

Nausea is uneasiness of the stomach with a feeling that retching or vomiting might follow. Vomiting is the forcible emptying of the stomach contents through the esophagus and mouth. Vomiting may occur as single or repeated spasms which the body uses to empty the stomach. Unfortunately, vomiting may continue as dry heaves even after the stomach is empty if the stimulus is strong enough. In projectile vomiting, the stomach contents are ejected in a forcible stream that may extend for several feet.

Complications

Nausea and vomiting may lead to serious dehydration and possibly malnutrition if prolonged. Dehydration may require intravenous fluids if the person is unable to keep liquids down for more than a day.

Finding the Homeopathic Medicine

- Ipecac is the first medicine to think of for strong nausea and vomiting.
- Use Bismuth or phosphorus when the vomiting is primarily of liquids, and they are vomited after becoming warm in the stomach.
- Nux vomica should be considered when the vomiting comes on from emotional stress, especially anger and frustration, and it is difficult for the person to vomit.
- Phosphorus can be considered for vomiting blood and for vomit that looks like coffee grounds, in a friendly, open, sympathetic person who desires cold drinks but vomits them.

- Tabacum is the best for nausea and vomiting from motion, like seasickness.
- Veratrum album is useful for a combination of nausea, vomiting, and diarrhea, especially if the person is cold but desires cold and sour foods such as lemons and pickles.

Self Care and Home Remedies

- Get some fresh air
- Eat small amounts of food frequently.
- Eat Saltine crackers to help relieve the nausea.
- Eat bland foods such as broth, rice, and pasta.
- Tea and toast are usually well tolerated.
- Drink clear fluids if you can keep them down.
- Sip ginger root tea to help relieve nausea. Use a one quarter inch slice of ginger root boiled in a cup of water for fifteen minutes.
- Stimulate stomach an acupressure point in the soft place below the knee and to the outside of the leg where the tibia and fibula bones meet, to relieve nausea. Use firm rotary pressure on the spot for a few seconds. Repeat when needed.

Stomach and Acute Abdominal Pain

Stomach and abdominal pain can range from mild discomfort to incapacitating pain. The causes are highly variable and include indigestion, gas, appendicitis, gall bladder inflammation, liver problems, menstrual cramping, acute gastroenteritis, ectopic pregnancy, miscarriage, cancer, and anxiety, as well as a number of other causes.

2

KIDNEY /URINARY BLADDER AND JOINT DISORDERS

Bladder Infections

Bladder infections are caused by microorganisms that colonize the bladder in susceptible patients. Bladder infections may have no apparent symptoms even though bacteria can be cultured from the urine. Symptoms may also occur with no apparent infection.

Symptoms

The most common symptoms are urgent desire to urinate, frequent urination, bladder pain, low back pain, and burning pain before, during or after urination. Bladder infections occur most commonly in women following sexual intercourse, especially with a new partner. Bladder infections can also occur after waiting too long without urinating or going too long without drinking liquids. Catheterization is a common source of bladder infections in hospitals and nursing homes. Bladder infections often come on with sudden severity, but can progress gradually.

Complications

There is risk of bladder infections ascending up the ureter to cause acute pyelonephritis, a serious infection of the kidneys. Pain along the sides of the mid-back along with urinary frequency, urgency, and pain is indicative of a kidney infection and requires immediate treatment.

Finding the Homeopathic Medicine

- The most common medicines for bladder infections are Cantharis and Staphysagiria.
- Give of Apis if the pain is mostly stinging and burning, swelling, the last drops feel scalding, and the urine will not come out easily.
- Give Cantharis if blood in the urine is prominent or the pain is excruciating. Cantharis has the most extreme bladder symptoms.
- If the major symptom is frequent, intense urging with severe pain, give Mercurius corrosivus.
- Sarsaparilla is a common medicine for women's bladder infections.
- If the major symptom is burning in the urethra at the close of urination, give Sarsaparilla. If it doesn't work, look at Staphysagria or Cantharis.
- If the bladder infection comes on after sex, take Staphysagria first.

Self Care and Home Remedies

- Drink as much water as possible.
- Urinate whenever you have the urge.
- Avoid horseback riding or other activities that put pressure on the urethra and bladder.
- Take bladder herbs such as Oregon grape, Buschu, Pipsissewa, and Uva ursi every two hours until symptoms

improve. The dosage will depend on whether it is a tea, capsule, or tincture.

- If citrus fruits aggravate your bladder, avoid them.
- Prevention include drinking liquids frequently and urinating as soon as possible after you feel the urge and after sex.

Joint Disorders

Back Pain

Pain in the back may be caused by a strain or sprain, by misalignment of the spinal vertebrae, or by pelvic bones causing pressure on neves. Back tension and spasms may also be caused by emotional states such as anger or fear.

Symptoms

Pain is present in the affected part of the back. The low back and neck are the most common sites of acute back pain. It is sometimes difficult and painful for the person to move or straighten up. Pain may be either dull or quite sharp, particularly when moving about. Muscles around the site of the pain are often in spasm.

Complications

Some acute back pain may be caused by a herniated vertebral disk. This type of pain usually extends into a limb and may be quite severe and accompanied by numbness. It is usually worse when sneezing, coughing or holding the breath, and bearing down. Acute pain in the mid-back may be caused by kidney stones or a kidney infection. Medical attention should be sought immediately for proper diagnosis, especially if fever is present or the pain is excruciating.

Finding the Homeopathic Medicine

- Give Arnica for sore, bruised back pain after an injury or trauma.
- Arnica is used before and after back surgery to promote healing.
- Bryonia is the best medicine when the main symptom is pain that is made worse by moving.
- Hypericum is good for direct injuries to the spine or neves, with shooting pain.
- Give Rhus toxicodendron when the pain is made worse by overexertion and getting wet, and better by limbering up and moving around.

Self Care and Home Remedies

- When the injury first occurs, apply an ice pack if there is swelling or inflammation.
- After twelve to twenty four hours, apply moist heat to the area.
- Take a hot bath with one cup of Epsom salts added. Whirlpool baths or hot tubs are also good.
- Rest in bed in a comfortable position.
- Acupuncture, chiropractic, osteopathy, physical therapy, Bowen therapy (an Australian bodywork technique), massage, or other bodywork techniques are often helpful if homoeopathy is not producing immediate results.

Sprains and Strains

A sprain is an injury to the muscles, tendons, and ligaments–the connective tissues that surround joints. Sprains and strains results from twisting, turning, moving, of falling in such a way as to cause an injury. They can also result from overuse.

Symptoms

Pain (mild to severe) and stiffness are the main symptoms of sprains and strains.

Complications

In cases of severe pain, it is helpful to seek immediate attention and, if appropriate, obtain an X ray to make sure there are no fractures or dislocations.

Finding the Homeopathic Medicine

- The best medicine to give first for sprains and strains is Arnica.
- If the pain is worse from any motion, give Bryonia.
- If the injured area is cold to the touch and the pain is better from cold applications, Ledum is the best medicine.
- If the main symptom is stiffness that is better from moving around and stretching, Rhus toxicodendron will be of benefit.
- If there is injury to ligaments or tendons without any clear picture that points to one of the other medicines, give Ruta.

Self Care and Home Remedies

- Put ice pack on the injured area. Previously sports medicine doctors used to recommend icing for the first twenty-four to forty-eight hours, then applying heat, but now many suggest continuing to apply ice pack to the injury. Ice reduces swelling and inflammation.
- Rest the injured area. If necessary immobilize it, including using crutches.
- Wrap the injured part with an elastic bandage.

- Apply an ointment, cream, or gel of topical Arnica.
- Soak in an Epsom salt tub or foot bath to help reduce swelling.

Sciatica

Sciatica is pain along the distribution of the sciatic nerve in the back of the leg, resulting from inflammation and compression of the nerve at its root near the spine, in the buttocks, or in the pelvis. The nerve compression in the spine often comes from a herniated intervertebral disk.

Symptoms

Pain begins in the back or pelvis and radiates down the leg partially or all the way to the foot. The pain may be quite severe and accompanied by numbness and tingling. It is usually worse when sneezing, coughing, or holding the breath and bearing down.

Complications

The disk problem can get worse if lifting and straining are not done properly, increasing the sciatic pain sometimes to the point of incapacitation.

Finding the Homeopathic Medicine

- If there is twitching and spasms in a person who seems intoxicated, think of Agaricus.
- If the sciatica comes on after anger or being offended, give Colocynthis.
- If the sciatica is on the right side and has pain along with numbness, give Gnaphhalium.
- If the sciatica is from an injury to the spine, Hypericum is probably the right medicine.

- If the person wakes in the early morning with the sciatica, give Kali iodatum.
- If other symptoms are left sided, but the sciatica is right sided, think of Lachesis.
- If the symptoms are worse from sitting and better from moving around, consider Rhus toxicodendron.
- If a herniated disk is definitely involved consider Tellurium, especially if the person has ringworm also.

Self Care and Home Remedies

- Apply moist heat to the low back and buttocks.
- Take a hot bath with one cup of Epsom salts added. Whirlpool baths or hot tubs are also good.
- Rest in bed in a comfortable position.
- The Bowen Therapeutic Technique, an Austrialian bodywork practice, is very useful for treating sciatica.
- Acupuncture, chiropractic, osteopathy, physical therapy, or massage may be helpful if homoeopathy is not producing immediate results.
- Take Calcium (1500mg) and Magnesium (750mg) daily to reduce muscle spasms.
- Arnica gel or oil is very helpful when applied locally to the area.

3

SKIN DISORDERS

Allergic Reactions

Allergic reactions can be mild or severe. They occur when the body is exposed to an allergen–a substance in the environment that causes an immune-system response. The response is triggered by the release of histamine from the mast cells, which are part of the immune system. Allergic reactions are caused by an immune-system response that is greater than is needed to respond to the presence of a foreign substance in the body.

Symptoms

Allergic symptoms include swelling, itching, redness, inflammation, sneezing, mucous discharges, hives or other skin rashes, asthma, and systemic shock, as seen in an anaphylactic response.

Complications

Anaphylactic shock and respiratory arrest: If the person has a severe reaction to an allergen, including significant itching and swelling of lymph nodes, swelling of the mucous membranes of the nose and ears, and difficult breathing due to constriction of the air passages, this is likely to be an anaphylactic response and requires emergency care. If untreated, anaphylaxis can be rapidly fatal.

Homoeopathic Medicine

- If the person's nose runs like a faucet with streaming eyes, give Allium cepa.

- If swelling and stinging pains are the prominent symptoms, consider Apis.
- If anxiety and restlessness are the most significant symptoms, think of Arsenicum.
- If symptoms occur after getting wet or over work, and stiffness and itching eruptions are present, give Rhustox.
- If the allergic reaction is to shellfish, or feels like stinging nettles or a burn, give Urtica urens.

Self Care and Home Remedies

- For shock: lie down, keep warm, drink fluids.
- For itching: Soak in a bathtub of warm water with one cup of baking soda or one cup of raw oatmeal.
- For swelling: ice pack or cold wet compresses.

Diaper Rash

Diaper rash is a skin irritation or infection which occurs when wet diapers stay in prolonged contact with the baby's skin.

Symptoms

The skin is moist, red and raw. Red spots or patches may indicate a yeast infection due to Candida. Bacterial infection may cause blistering and pus.

Complications

Diaper rash rarely causes anything other than local inflammation or infection. If a high fever is present without another obvious cause and the lymph glands in the groin are swollen, seek medical attention to rule out an infection in the blood stream.

Finding the Homoeopathic Medicine

Babies needing Hepar sulphuris are generally extremely chilly and very sensitive to uncovering. They have an infected diaper rash with pus that smells like rotten cheese.

Infants who need Graphites have diaper rash in the folds of the skin, which is dry, red, cracked, and very itchy, with a honey like discharge that crusts over.

Babies needing medorrhinum have a sharply demarcated red, sometimes shiny diaper rash often caused by Candida infection, called "thrush diaper rash."

Infants who need Sulphur have a red, dry, itchy diaper rash around the anus that is worse from getting overheated and from a warm bath.

Self Care and Home Remedies

Let the baby go without diapers whenever possible.

- Change diapers whenever they become wet or soiled.
- Cleanse the area with very mild soap and water.
- Dry the area carefully with a hairdryer on the lowest heat.
- Apply Calendula cream after every diaper change until diaper rash is gone.
- Cornstarch may be useful on the skin as a drying powder.
- Use all cotton diapers instead of rubber pants.

Frostbite

Frostbite is the freezing of a part of the body from exposure to cold.

Symptoms

The affected body part becomes cold, hard, and white as it is actually frozen, and is usually not painful until it warms up again.

The part may become red, itching and throbbing on rewarming, and blistering may occur.

Complications

If severe, frostbite may lead to gangrene, in which the tissue becomes black and eventually sloughs off. The limb may require amputation as a result of the gangrene. If the frostbitten area is black, seek medical attention immediately.

Finding the Homeopathic Medicine

- Agaricus is always the first medicine to consider for frostbite.
- In mild frostbite with splinter like pains, Nitric acid is the best choice.
- If there is bluish red discoloration, itching, and pain, especially in the feet, consider Pulsatilla.
- If the frostbitten area feels worse from rubbing and the person has restless legs, give Zincum metallicum.

Self Care and Home Remedies

- Do not apply ice or snow to the frozen part.
- Rewarm the part as soon as possible, preferably with circulating warm water or contact with warmth, but not with excessive heat.

Hives

Hives appear on the skin as part of an allergic reaction to a food or an environmental allergen such as pollen, dust mites or wool. Hives may also occur due to exercise or from becoming cold.

Symptoms

Hives are red, raised welts that are often quite itchy, hot, and swollen.

Complications

In a serious case of acute hives, anaphylaxis(characterized by intense itching, swelling, and difficulty in breathing due to constriction of the bronchioles) can be life-threatening and requires emergency medical attention. Hives may become chronic or may occur repeatedly if the allergen that causes the body to react is not eliminated.

Finding the Homeopathic Medicine

- If there is tremendous swelling, give Apis first.
- For hives due to bee stings, give Apis.
- If itching is the main symptom and the person is very restless, give Rhus toxicodendron.
- If the hives sting and there is not significant swelling, consider Urtica urens.

Self Care and Home Remedies

- For itching: soak in a bathtub of warm water with one cup of baking soda or one cup of raw oatmeal.
- For swelling: ice pack or cold wet compresses.
- Take 500 mg Vitamin C twice a day.

Cold Sores

Cold sores are caused by a virus, Herpes Simplex Virus I, which remains dormant in the nerve roots around the mouth. Episodes of outbreaks occur whenever stress levels are too high and the immune system is not strong enough to keep the virus in check. Exposure to the sun can also cause a recurrence.

Symptoms

Single or multiple blisters, which may be as large as a dime, usually occur on or around the lips. The blisters are often accompanied by swelling and are usually quite painful. Numbness and tingling may occur before the blisters appear, as well as fatigue.

Complications

Cold sores will usually disappear on their own in one to two weeks. There are usually no complications, although scarring may occur in some cases.

Finding the Homeopathic Medicine

- Natrum muriaticum is the most frequently used medicine for cold sores.
- For cold sores that come on from exposure to the sun in a sensitive person who easily gets her feelingshurt, the most common medicine is Natrum muriaticum.
- Cold sores that burn in a chilly,anxious, restless person may require Arsenicum album.
- People needing Hepar sulphuris are generally extremely chilly and their sensitivity to the pain of the cold sores seems out of proportion.
- Cold sores that occur after exertion or exposure to cold, damp weather usually respond to Rhus toxicodendron.

Self Care and Home Remedies

- Lysine: 500mg three times a day.
- Vitamin C: 1000mg three times a day.

  Beta carotene: 50,000IU a day.

  Zinc: 30 mg a day.
- One part Calendula tincture mixed with three parts water applied with a cotton swab three times a day.

Contact Dermatitis

Poison ivy, oak, and sumag cause a contact dermatitis. Some people are highly sensitive to these plants, and some show no sensitivity. Poison ivy and sumac are more common in the eastern part of the United States, and poison oak in the west. The oil of these plants can be spread around the body by touch. It can also cause a severe reaction if the plants are burned and the smoke inhaled.

Symptoms

An extremely itchy, red, blistering rash that causes great discomfort and annoyance, and often takes more than a week to heal. The blisters ooze and crust over before drying up.

Complications

These skin rashes are usually self limiting and cause no long term effects. The homeopathic proving of poison ivy suggests that arthritis could be a long term complication if the skin rash is suppressed by external applications such as hydrocortisone cream.

Finding the Homeopathic Medicine

- Anacardium is often the most effective medicine for poison ivy, oak, and sumac.
- Croton tiglium can be used if the skin feels incredibly itchy and hidebound, and there is gushing diarrhea.
- Rhus toxicodendron is the most available medicine, and will often work.

Self Care and Home Remedies

- Be careful not to spread the rash by scratching it, then scratching an unaffected area.

- Wash the area with mild soap and water and cover with sterile gauze, if needed, to keep it clean.
- Calendula lotion is soothing to the rash and irritated skin.
- Cold wet applications can help the rash feel better, especially cold comfrey root tea.
- Oatmeal bath: Use Aveno or place one cup of finely blended dry Oatmeal in the bath to sooth itching.
- If secondary infection from scratching occurs, cleanse with Calendula soap and water and apply Calendula gel or lotion.

Skin Infections: Boils, Folliculitis, and Carbuncles

Boils, folliculitis, and carbuncles are skin infections, usually associated with Staphylococcus aureus bacteria.

Symptoms

Folliculitis is an infection of the hair follicules with redness, tenderness, and swelling. Boils, also called furuncles, are more advanced skin infections which form a large eruption that discharges bloody pus. Boils are most common on the neck, face, breasts, and buttocks. Boils can be quite painful and especially tender to pressure. A collection of boils that forms one large infected area penetrating deeper into the tissue is called a carbuncle. Carbuncles are common at the base of the neck. They may be accompanied by fatigue and fever. They are slow to heal, slough off tissue with blood and pus, and can cause scarring.

Complications

Skin infections can lead to a serious systemic blood infection called septicemia. The symptoms of septicemia are a high fever and organ damage. Septicemia can be fatal. Red streaks extending from the infected area toward the heart are a red flag for septicemia and indicate a need for immediate medical attention.

Finding the Homeopathic Medicine

- For crusty, oozing, black eruptions, give Anthracinum.
- For infections with small, red, ulcerated pimples and burning pains, consider Arsenicum album, especially if the person is nervous and restless.
- If the person screams when you examine the infected area, give Hepar sulphuris.
- If the infected area is bluish purple and left- sided, consider Lachesis.
- For infections with bad smelling discharges and perspiration and bad breath, Mercurius is the first thought.
- For infections due to an ingrown nail, think first of Silica.

Self Care and Home Remedies

- Hot, moist packs can be helpful for folliculitis and boils to bring the infection to a head.
- An echinacea and goldenseal combination (two dropperfuls of tincture in water three times a day or six capsules a day) is useful to stimulate the immune system to fight infection.
- Give Vitamin A (25,000 IU a day) or beta carotene(50,000 IU a day).
- Give Vitamin C (1000mg three times a day).
- Give Zinc (30mg a day).

4

MALE & FEMALE DISORDERS

MALE DISORDERS

Impotency

Why Impotence Shouldn't Be Ignored

The percentage of men suffering from E.D. (Erectile Dysfunction i.e. Impotency) is very high in our society, but for obvious reasons they don't come forward and continue to suffer, despite having strong sexual desires. Imagine what it must be like not being able to have physical relations for 12 to 15 years !

Anyway, more and more research and articles and support groups are required to address this problem, which has assumed massive proportions. After all, the fitness of our apparatus is very necessary for keeping the other half of the society happy!

The Culprit in Your Case

After taking a detailed history with special reference etc. medical problems and lifestyle habits, your andrologist/urologist will administer these tests:

- The Nocturnal Penile Turnescense Test in which a computer is attached to the penis at night, to check for erection.
- Intra Penile Injections increase the blood flow to the penis and result in an erection which is observed and rate.

- A Penile Ultra Sound Colour Doppler visualizes the blood vessels in the penis.

MIND OR MATTER?

It is Psychological if

- you wake up with an early morning or middle-of-the-night erection,
- you have had satisfactory interactive intercourse,
- you masturbate perfectly well, and
- your problem occurred suddenly.

It is Physical if

- your erection is feeble and does not strengthen even while you sleep, wake up in the morning, or masturbate
- you fail again and again, and
- the onset is gradual.

Irksome Illnesses

By far the most common illnesses that cause impotence is diabetes; over half of all older diabetics have or will have erectile difficulties; 20% of hypertensive can suffer, too.

Other culprits are high cholesterol, spinal injury, pelvic surgery, excessive drinking and smoking which damage the blood vessels.

Incidentally the latest research shows that if you suffer from vascular erectile dysfunction, it is wise to have a cardiac check up, because a link has been established between furred arteries of the penis and faculty arteries of the heart.

With added medical awareness, prescribed drugs such as antihistamines and antidepressants are being held responsible for only 10% of the cases.

Harmon imbalances are even rarer, account for a more 1 %.

Something For Everyone

Treatments for impotence are available for every age, condition, need, preference or social situation.

Homoeopathic Medicines

Lycopodium

It is the most famous homeopathic medicine. Famous serologist of U.S.A. Dr. Nash M.D. says that if taken in proper dose this drug not only makes youth robust filled with abundant semen, it even revitalize the sexual potency of the old persons. The effect of the medicine is not temporary but permanent one, hence it should be administered in fixed intervals of time. This medicine is available in various potencies, from 200 to 10000 or even of one lakh potency. The higher the potency the better would be the results. But it is advisable that these medicines should be taken after proper medical advice. Or else they create quite serious complications. This medicine is especially recommended for those strayed youth who ruin their sexual potency by constant use of their male organ. In fact this medicine should be taken by increasing its potency gradually. The medicine of 200 potency should be given on empty stomach to the patient and the next dose of higher potency after one full week. The same way the potency should be increased from 1000 to the dose of the desired potency when the affliction is cured.

Phosphoric Acid

It is also a wonder homoeopathic drug to cure sexual weakness. The constant malpractice result in the patient's face becoming pale and sallow, eyes sunken in the sockets and constant complaints of pain in the waist. The afflicted person's semen also becomes very thin and often passes out with urine while passing stool. This medicine is also good for those patients afflicted with diabetes. It not only enhances the physical power of the patient but makes him very strong mentally also. This medicine is to be administered mixed with three to five drops of mother tincture diluted with 25 to 30 gms. of water. Ask the patient to have the medicine before taking his meal. Phosphoric acid is a powerful drug and should not be administered on empty stomach.

Avenazativa

The cautious use of this celebrated medicine administered mixed with five to six drops of mother tincture is an unfailing remedy for all the sexual weakness. A timid listless boy turns into a robust man by the use of this medicine. It not only strengthens the user's body but increases the efficiency of his mental faculties.

Caution

All these medicines are to be taken after proper medical advice. Don't rush to take them without consulting some good homoeopathic physician. Other good remedies are caladium, conium, staphysagria and selenium.

FEMALE DISORDERS

Dysnenoshoea(Mensturral Cramps)

Finding the Homoeopathic Medicine

- If there is heavy, bright red bleeding, gushing and throbbing pain, look first at Belladonna.
- If the pain is lessened by heat and pressure, think first of Magnesia phosphorica, then of Colocynthis.

- For pain is very intense and the woman is terribly angry and inconsolable, look at Chamomilla.
- If the woman feels better when drawing her knees up to her chest, give Colocynthis.
- If the pain began after anger, think of Nux vomica, Colocynthis, and Belladonna.
- If the pain came on after too much alcohol or rich food, give Nux vomica.

Self Care and Home Remedies

- Alternating hot and cold sitz baths: soak in tub of moderately hot water for five minutes, then in a tub of cold water up to the navel with knees bent for one minute. Alternate two to three times.
- Walking stretching and other physical exercise can sometimes help.
- For muscle cramps, Calcium and Magnesium can help.
- Take Viburnum tincture: one half teaspoon every hour, up to six doses. The dosage for capsules depends on the specific product.
- A heating pad is often helpful.
- Castor oil packs to the abdomen with a heating pad can sometimes relieve discomfort
- Avoid caffeine and salt premenstrually.

PAIN REDUCES PLEASURE

After my children were born, I have not enjoyed sex at all. I am protected against getting pregnant again so I feel that's not a problem. Also, I enjoyed sex a lot before children. Sometimes I think its all in my head, that if I could let myself enjoy it, I wouldn't feel any pain; yet I know there's something wrong. My gynaecologist has not been able to figure anything out.

This kind of report typifies a woman who is eager for a sexual experience but is finding each encounter to be more and more negative because of the intense pain she experiences during each sexual act. Pain during intercourse is technically called dyspareunia. It has a number of different sources. Whatever the source, when pain is experienced sexual enjoyment will be greatly reduced if not eliminated altogether.

Pain and the New Bride

For the new bride who is a virgin it is not surprising if there is a small amount of pain. Most women experience at least a little. This can be due to the opening in the hymen being tight and small. In the great majority of situations it is due to a combination of new, excitement and anxiety which prevents the woman from relaxing. When the necessary physical changes do not take place (the opening up and laying flat of the majora lips, plus lubrication), then entry is going to be more difficult and pain more intense. Entry under these conditions increases the pain and reduces the possibility of pleasure. Once the woman feels pain, tension is likely to set in. This tension will inhibit arousal and block any kind of release. While many couples begin in this way they usually get past the sequence quite quickly. But the sequence can be avoided to begin with.

If you are an engaged couple or if you counsel engaged couples, attending to a few small details will reduce much of the anxiety and potential for pain. First six weeks to two months before the wedding date the woman should be examined by gynaecologist or qualified general practitioner. In this experience the doctor should be able to communicate to her whether her physical anatomy is normal and whether there are any particular barriers of which she should be aware. The couple and the physician should discuss birth control methods.

In the weeks before the marriage, every time the bride-to-be takes a bath she should use her fingers to stretch the hymen until she can insert three fingers into the vagina and pull it apart slightly. This stretching procedure will prepare the vagina for entry and will also help the woman become familiar with some of the sensations of having the vagina stretched. As the wedding comes closer this might be done several times a day.

The couple should be encouraged to take along a lubricant that is not sticky (not Vaseline). K-Y jelly or Lubrifax are recommended for genital use. For use over the whole body as well as genitally, a nonallergic lotion without lanolin such as Allercreme is good. The couple should plan to use the lubricant for all entry experiences, whether they think they need it or not. The lubricant protects the woman in case she dries up during the excitement. It also provides a distraction from the focus on the entry. A small amount of lubricant should be applied to the head and ridge of the penis and to the opening of the vagina.

A final word of instruction to the new bride and groom is to move slowly. No matter how many times they tell themselves to proceed slowly they will still most likely move ahead too quickly. If a couple can plan to move into their first experience with a great deal of gentleness, patience, ease, and relaxation, they are most likely to create a positive beginning to a life of loving.

Stress Bring Pain

All of us show our tension in our own unique way. Some women, as they experience tension surrounding the sexual experience, will tend to tighten up their genital muscles involuntarily. In fact, they may not even be aware that the tensing is happening. Since this is counterproductive to a fulfilling and releasing sexual experience, it is not surprising that these women end up frustrated. But even more than the frustration as a result of the tension, they may experience pain. For example, if the tightening occurs before entry it may cause pain upon entry. Sharp, spasmodic contractions after entry may also cause pain. The extreme form of this tension is called vaginismus.

Vaginimus is the involuntary tightening of the muscles in the outer side of the vagina which prevents the insertion of the penis. This contraction can be so severe that it is impossible to insert even your small finger. It can become a permanent state rather than just occurring as a result of the initiation of sex play. Because it is impossible for the man to enter, vaginismus is easily identified. Should this be your situation, consult a gynaecologist immediately and specifically explain your situation. If he or she is not familiar with the usual treatment procedures ask for a referral either to another physician or to a sex therapist. This professional must be competent to guide you in the use of a series of dilators which are graduated in size and designed to eliminate these involuntary spasms. Be encouraged that this condition is extremely responsive to treatment in a relatively brief period of time. However, there should be some attempt also to understand the events leading to the vaginismus so that this pattern will not be repeated.

Another source of pain due to tension occurs with lack of release. When a woman does not experience an orgasm, she may sense some painful sensations in the lower abdominal area and the lower back. As she has become aroused the whole reproductive system, including the vaginal area and the uterus has become congested with blood in preparation for the orgasmic release. The contractions of the orgasm are designed to release it's congestion so that the blood which has fined the cavities can be drained. When there is an orgasm this process provides a great deal of pleasure. When the woman does not experience release, the whole pelvic area remains engorged, which may cause chronic pain. This pain is usually not intense, but is a dull, throbbing ache similar to lower back pain. The difference is that it feels like it is further inside the body. Obviously the best remedy for this pain is for a woman to allow herself to experience orgasm. Consulting a physician or therapist it is crucial to identify when the pain occurs and thus determine if it is the result of lack of orgasmic release.

Physically Based Pain

Infections and irritations will obviously reduce pleasure. Whether the infection is in the external genitalia, causing pain during clitoral stimulation, or is inside the vagina, causing pain during intercourse, it will hinder freedom and enjoyment. Any kind of infection should immediately be dealt with by a physician. Sexual activity should be limited according to the instruction of the physician. Sometimes an infection provides the opportunity for the couple to focus on the rest of the body for those often bypassed, special pleasures. Just because there is an infection does not mean the couple should abstain from all sexual activity. If it is comfortable for both, the man can be stimulated to orgasm at the end of a total body experience without ever having contact with the woman's genitals.

Irritations are troublesome because there is no specific identifiable disease present. Yet an irritated vaginal opening or vaginal barrel can cause as much distress and pain during love-making as an infection. The best antidote to irritation is the generous use of a lubricant. Some women experience a thinning of the vaginal walls. Sometimes this happens with age, particularly around the time of menopause because of a reduction of estrogen. If the walls of your vagina are thinning, again consult a physician to determine the cause and then always use a lubricant to reduce friction. Even if the walls of the vagina are becoming thin, pleasurable activity need not cease.

Pain can also be the result of tears either in the opening of the vagina or small cuts (fissures) inside the vagina itself. Tears in the hymen usually cause pain on entry. Some women can identify pain at a very specific spot inside the vagina. Their report usually goes something like this: "It feels as if it is in the lower left-hand corner about an inch inside the vagina and it hurts exactly the same way every time. I feel I can even reach in and put my finger on it". When the pain is this specific, it is usually not the result of tension or the thinning of the vaginal walls but rather the result of a small tear inside the vagina. Because of continued sexual activity and the environment, healing is slow. When consulting a physician be sure to identify the exact location of the pain. Show the doctor so that he can carefully warn it and determine the nature of the problem. As a rule these tears can be treated with an ointment.

Some women report pain only during deep thrusting. There are three main sources of this kind of pain. The most commonly reported discomfort is the result of a lipped or retroverted uterus. When the muscles that suspend the uterus are weakened, the uterus drops so that the cervix, the opening to the uterus falls into the upper end of the vagina. As deep thrusting occurs the penis strikes the cervix, causing sharp, stabbing pain. It may cause a woman to cry out. Relief can be found immediately by a slight shift in position. For many women a small pillow or folded towel under the lower back (if she is under the man) will shift the uterus enough so that deep thrusting can be enjoyed.

Other internal pathologies such as endometriosis or a misplaced IUD can also cause pain upon deep thrusting.

Finally, there may be pain as an outgrowth of trauma from childbirth. One such pain occurs in the sensitive scars from the episiotomy, the incision that is made between the vagina and the rectum to assist the birth process. There also may be tears in the ligaments that hold the uterus in place, in the vaginal wall or around the opening of the vagina. Tears are more likely to occur with a difficult birth. For those resuming sexual activity after the birth of a child I would issue the same encouragement given to the newly married couple: move carefully and slowly, haste will only hurt; be generous with the lubricant.

Managing Pain

Whenever you experience pain, the first thing you should do is talk about it with your husband. Never grit your teeth and bear it. Define exactly where the pain is located and when in the love-making process it occurs. Even before you get to the physician you may be able to avoid the situations that cause the pain if you guide the penis for entry and shift positions to make adjustments. Except for pain from deep thrusting, lubrication will almost always reduce some of the intensity, even if it is from an infection. Then, discover what is pleasurable and focus on that for the time being. Avoiding entry for a few love-making sessions may be necessary. It is important not to continue the activity that triggers the pain. Whenever a negative sensation like pain is associated with a pleasurable activity like sexual play or intercourse, the pleasurable event will begin to take on the negative feelings. Even after the physical reason for the pain has healed, a woman may continue to tense up or avoid the sexual activity that was linked with the pain. Her pulling away and tightening up has become a conditioned response. Sometimes the pain will continue because of the tension. In dealing with this, use the same approach as you would for any emotional hesitancy or avoidance. Begin gradually, letting the woman take the lead until the tension concerning the pain has been reduced.

An increasing number of women, particularly young women, are reporting pain during intercourse. If you are among these, seek help after talking about it with your partner. Pain does not have to be tolerated. In fact, pain cannot be allowed to continue if you are going to enjoy sexual pleasure.

Morning Sickness

Morning sickness occurs most commonly in the first three months of pregnancy, but may persist in some cases until the baby is born. It is commonly experienced in the morning, but may last throughout the day or come at different times.

Symptoms

Terrible nausea with aversion to the sight and smell of food are usual symptoms. Vomiting may be pronounced, with inability to keep most food and beverages down.

Complications

Apart from the discomfort and inconvenience, the main complication of prolonged morning sickness is malnutrition and failure of the mother to gain appropriate weight, with subsequent low birth weight and congenital health problems for the child. Hyperemesis gravidarum–severe uncontrollable vomiting in pregnancy, often associated with liver disease–may cause dehydration and acidosis, requiring hospitalization and intravenous fluids.

Finding the Homeopathic Medicine

- The most common medicines for morning sickness are Sepia and Colchicum.
- When aversion to the smell of food is strongest, consider Colchicum first.
- For the worst vomiting, use Ipecac, and for the most deathly nausea, use Tabacum.
- When aversion to sex is a strong symptom, consider Sepia or Kreosotum.
- Sepia is for conditions that are made much better by vigorous exercise or dancing, which separates it from the motion sickness medicines such as Tabacum and Cocculus; the latter two are appropriate for conditions that are made much worse by motion.
- Veratrum is the medicine if the woman is very cold, has vomiting and diarrhea and desires fruit, ice, and sour foods such as pickles or lemons.

Self Care and Home Remedies

- Eat small amounts of food frequently.
- Eat before getting up in the morning.
- Eat Saltine crackers to help relieve the nausea.
- Eat bland foods such as broth, rice, and pasta.
- Tea and toast are usually well tolerated.

- Sipping ginger root tea can help relieve nausea. Use a one quarterinch slice of ginger root boiled in a cup of water for fifteen minutes.
- Many herbs, such as pennyroyal, need to be avoided during pregnancy.
- Stimulating stomach, an acupressure point in the soft place below the knee and to the outside of the leg where the tibia and fibula bones meet, often relieves nausea. Use firm rotary pressure on the spot for a few seconds. Repeat when needed.

Thrush

Thrush is a yeast infection of the mucous membranes inside the mouth. It is common in infants, people who have been treated with antibiotics, and people with compromised immune systems, as in AIDS.

Symptoms

There are creamy white patches on the tongue or the mucous membranes of the mouth that can be scraped off.

Complications

None, unless the thrush continues for a long time and turns into a systemic yeast infection.

Finding the Homeopathic Medicine

- By far the most common medicine for thrush is Borax, especially if there are also canker sores.
- If there is bad smelling breath, perspiration, and body odor, give Mercurius.
- If the tongue burns and has a thick furry coating, consider Sulphur.

Self Care and Home Remedies

- If the nursing baby had thrush, the mother should also be treated if she has a breast infection.
- Acidophilus or unsweetened yogurt can help reestablish healthy intestinal flora.
- Avoid eating anything sweet, since yeast thrives on sugar.
- The most common treatment for thrush in many parts of the world is topical gentian violet, but it stains and is generally unnecessary due to the effectivenenss of homoeopathy.

Vaginitis

Vaginitis is an inflammation of the mucous membranes of the vagina. It may be caused by a viral, bacterial, trichomonal, or yeast infection, or by sexual intercourse, douching, or other irritants such as spermicides, chemicals, or a foreign body in the vagina. Atrophic vaginitis occurs in women past menopause, resulting from a decrease in estrogen levels.

Symptoms

Vaginal discharge is often the main complaint. It may be thick or thin, odorless or offensive. There may also be redness of the vaginal lips and itching, swelling or pain of the vulva, labia and vagina. The intensity varies greatly.

Complications

A culture of the vaginal discharge should be taken to find out the cause of the infection. If gonorrhea, chlamydia, or syphilis are found to be the cause, the diagnosis must be reported to the local public health department and immediate medical attention is required. These three infections are often asymptomatic in women and, if untreated, may lead to infertility.

Finding the Homeopathic Medicine

- For vaginitis with terrible itching during pregnancy, give Caladium.
- For vaginal discharges that are terribly abrasing and acrid, give Kreosotum.
- For vaginitis with a yellowish green creamy discharge in a gentle woman who cries as she tells you about it, Pulsatilla will probably work.
- If the discharge smells strongly like fish brine, look at Sanicula.
- If the symptoms occur during menopause and are accompanied by a lack of sex drive, constipation, and irritability, Sepia will be helpful.

Self Care and Home Remedies

- The easiest and most effective suggestion: insert one capsule of boric acid into the vagina in the morning, and one capsule of acidophilus at bedtime, for five days. Stop during the menstrual period.
- Douche with one tablespoon of white vinegar in a pint of warm water daily for five days. Insert one tablespoon of unsweetened, live culture yogurt after each douche.
- If the vaginitis is just on the labia and vulva and is caused by yeast, apply a preparation of half vinegar and half water topically.
- Some women insert a clove of garlic, wrapped in cheesecloth or gauze, vaginally for yeast infections.
- If there is rawness externally not due to yeast, Calendula cream topically can be helpful.

- Insert Vitamin E suppositories into the vagina for vaginal dryness.
- Occasionally, one tablespoon of baking soda in a quart of water works better as a douche than acidifying treatments such as vinegar or boric acid.

5

EYE-EAR-NOSE-THROAT DISORDERS

Eye Disorders

Stye

A stye is an infection of a sweat or oil gland in the eyelid.

Symptoms

The first symptoms are usually pain, redness, swelling, and tenderness of the edge of the eyelid, followed by the appearance of a small, round, tender, hardened area. Tears, sensitivity to light, and a feeling of a foreign body in the eye may follow.

Complications

Complications are rare, but styes are often recurrent.

Finding the Homeopathic Medicine

- If the styes are pus filled and sensitive to drafts, give Hepar sulphuris.
- For styes of the right eye with lots of dryness, look at Lycopodium.
- If the main symptom is profuse, thick, yellowish discharge from the eye, give Pulsatilla.
- For dry, painful eyes in a woman who never gets angry, give Staphysagria.
- If the edges of the lids are red, burning, itchy, and irritated, give Sulphur.

Self Care and Home Remedies

- Keep the eye clean.
- Place compresses soaked in hot water on the eyelid for ten minutes several times a day to bring the stye to a head and allow it to drain.
- Give Vitamin C (500mg two times a day) for immune support.

Conjunctivitis

Conjunctivitis, also known as pink eye, is an acute inflammation of the conjunctiva of the eye, which is a thin protective lining of the eyelids and eyeball. It is caused by bacterial or viral infection or an allergic sensitivity to an irritant.

Symptoms

The eye appears red and bloodshot, and there is often lots of watering and a clear or purulent (pus) discharge, depending on whether the infection is viral or bacterial. The eyelids are usually swollen. Intense itching occurs with allergic conjunctivitis. The eye feels irritated and painful, and there is a burning sensation or a feeling that something is in the eye.

Complications

Conjunctivitis may become chronic or may damage the eye if left untreated.

Finding the Homeopathic Medicine

- If the main symptom is puffy swelling of the eyelids, give Apis.
- For conjunctivitis in newborns, think of Argentum nitricum.

- When fever, redness, and throbbing pain are prominent, Belladonna is the medicine.
- If the main symptom is excessive, irritating tears, give Euphrasia.
- If the discharge is thick, creamy, and yellow green in a whiny, moody person, give Pulsatilla.
- If burning in the eyes is prominent in a lazy, philosophical egoist, give Sulphur.

Self Care and Home Remedies

- Apply a clean washcloth that has been dipped in cold water and wrung out over the eyes. Replace it when it gets warm.
- Rub the hands together vigorously and place over the closed eyes for one minute.
- Do not touch the other eye after you have touched the infected eye, to avoid spreading the infection.
- Use sterile Euphrasia eyedrops to soothe the eyes, a few drops in each eye after you have touched the infected eye, to avoid spreading the infection.
- Use sterile Euphrasia eyedrops to soothe the eyes, a few drops in each eye several times a day.
- Dissolve one fourth teaspoon of salt in one cup of water.
- Use three cotton balls soaked in the water to swipe the edge of the eyelids from inside to outside. Discard after using once. Repeat four times a day.
- Take beta carotene (50,000 IU per day) or Vitamin A (25,000 IU per day). Take Vitamin C (500mg, two times per day).

Ear Disorders

Ear Infection

Ear infections may be either internal or external. Otitis media, a middle ear infection, occurs behind the eardrum. Otitis externa, an outer ear infection, occurs in the ear canal outside the drum. Acute middle ear infections are associated with bacteria. Chronic middle ear inflammation may come from chronic bacterial infection or a buildup of fluid, usually caused by allergic reactions. Infants who are exposed to solid food and cow's milk too early may develop significant food allergies which are directly correlated with chronic ear infections. The allergies often begin right after the child is weaned from breast feeding.

Symptoms

Middle ear infections cause acute pain, a clogged or blocked sensation in the ear with some temporary loss of hearing, and bulging of the eardrum. More rarely, the eardrum can rupture, discharging pus and fluid into the ear canal. Chronic ear infections cause redness of the eardrum and pressure and blockage in the ears with some, usually reversible, hearing loss.

Complications

Following a rupture, the eardrum will usually repair itself, but may leave scarring. Chronic ear infections may cause hearing loss, which usually resolves when the fluid drains or disappears. In chronic middle ear inflammation with an allergic basis ("glue ear") antibiotics are inffective on a long term basis, and the causative allergic responses must be addressed. Even in acute ear infections, antibiotics may not shorten the course of illness. Conventional physicians often recommend surgical insertion of tubes into the eardrums to drain off the fluid, in order to prevent chronic hearing loss which may interfere with language development in young children.

Finding the Homeopathic Medicine

- If a child quickly develops an ear infection after playing in the cold air, she needs Aconite.
- If the child has intense, throbbing pain in the right ear, a bright red face, and a fever of 103°F or higher, give Belladonna.
- For fussy children whose ear infections are associated with teething Chamomilla is best.
- Children who scream with pain during an ear infection may need Hepar sulphuris, Belladonna, or Chamomilla.
- If memcurius is needed, there is likely to be bad breath, a coated tongue, excessive saliva, and bad smelling perspiration.
- Mild, moody children who cry easily and want to be held and caressed during an ear infection are likely to need Pulsatilla.
- If Silica is needed, there wil generally be a tendency to swollen glands, excessive bad smelling perspiration, and possibly a history of dental problems.

Self Care and Home Remedies

- Mullein garlic oil drops, three drops in the affected ear three times daily. Warm the oil bottle under the faucet first. Put a piece of cotton in the ear after inserting drops to prevent the oil from coming out. If there is a tendency for the infection to spread from one ear to the other, put the drops in both ears.
- Alternating hot and cold compresses to the affected ear.

- Beta-carotene: 50,000 units daily in acute cases; 25,000 units daily in chronic cases.
- It is often helpful to remove milk products from the diet, at least temporarily.
- Goat's milk is a good substitute for cow's milk.

Throat Disorders

Mumps

Mumps is a contagious viral infection of the parotid gland in the upper jaw, just below and in front of the ears and other salivary glands. Mumps usually occurs in children, but can be more serious in adults.

Symptoms

The primary symptoms are moderate to high fever with chills, and painful swelling of the parotid glands and other salivary glands with fatigue and loss of appetite.

Complications

In men past puberty, the main complication of mumps is painful inflammation of the testes which can, in rare cases, cause sterility. Meningoencephalitis, which resembles bacterial meningitis, is characterized by a headache, stiff neck, and, rarely, convulsions or a coma. Pancreatitis with nausea, vomiting, and pain in the abdomen sometimes occurs at the end of the first week of mumps, and gets completely better in about a week.

Finding the Homeopathic Medicine

- Mercurius is the most common medicine used for mumps
- Phytolacca is used to treat stony hard parotid glands with pain extending to on swallowing.

- Carbo vegetabils is used for mumps when exhaustion and bloating are prominent symptoms.
- Pulsatilla and Carbo vegetabilis are both used when mumps causes inflammation of the testes or breasts.
- Pulsatilla is appropriate when the child or adult is weepy and clingy with a lot of swelling in the testes or breasts.
- Less common medicines which help inflammation of the testes during or after mumps are Abrotanum and Jaborandi.
- Abrotannum is used to treat a large swollen parotid gland that goes down as the testes become swollen. It is given to irritable children with a failure to thrive.
- Jaborandi treats mumps with increased sweating and salivation, and parotid glands double their usual size. This medicine has been used to shorten the duration of the disease.

Self Care and Home Remedies

- Rest.
- Eat soft foods to reduce the need for chewing.
- Avoid spicy and sour foods and drinks, such as citrus fruit and other juices, which may cause pain by stimulating the salivary glands.
- Isolate the person with mumps to avoid spreading the infection to those who have not had it.
- Take Vitamin C, 500 mg two times daily for children four years or older.
- Use a carrot poultice to relieve swelling. Blend two to three carrots, place in a cloth or cheesecloth and apply under chin for two to eight hours.

Sore Throats

Pharyngitis is an inflammation of the pharynx or throat which is usually associated with a virus or, as in the case of a strep throat, a bacteria.

Symptoms

The most distressing symptom is usually a mild to severe pain in the throat, which may extend to the ears. There may be a simultaneous upper respiratory infection, bronchitis, or flu.

Complications

An untreated Group A Beta-hemolytic strep infection may lead to rheumatic fever or joint problems.

Finding the Homeopathic Medicine

- For throat pain of very rapid onset with a high fever, give Aconite or Belladonna.
- If it feels better from cold drinks, first look at Apis.
- If the main symptom is swelling, give Apis or Phytolacca.
- For very red sore throats, the best medicines are Belladonna and Apis.
- For a burning, right sided sore throat in a person with a bright red face and ear pain, give Belladonna.
- For right sided sore throats, think of Belladonna, Apis, Lycopodium, Phytolacca, and Mercurius iodatus flavus.
- The medicines to give for sore throats that have the most pain on swallowing are Lachesis, Hepar sulphuris, Belladonna, and Mercurius.
- For left sided sore throats, consider Lachesis first, then, more rarely, Mercurius iodatus ruber.

- The first medicine to consider for sore throats that start on the left then move to the right is Lachesis.
- For sore throats that begin on the right then go to the left, look at Lycopodium.
- If the sore throat feels better from warm drinks, think first of Lycopodium.

Self Care and Home Remedies

- Gargle with warm salt water three times a day.
- Gargle with one teaspoon of Calendula tincture in one cup of warm water.
- Suck on zinc lozenges. (Avoid any lozenges with menthol, camphor, or eucalyptus, since they interfere with homeopathic treatment.)
- Take Vitamin C (3000 mg a day) in divided doses of 500 mg. Cut the dose in half for a child and give a maximum of 250 mg to a baby.
- Take echinacea and goldenseal tincture in water (one half teaspoon every two hours, up to six doses a day).
- Avoid dairy products and sweets.
- Drink one to two glasses of fresh carrot juice per day.

Nose Disorders

Epistaxis

Nose-bleeds are simply spontaneous bleeding from the nose. They are caused by infections of the nose and sinuses, dryness and cracking of the nasal mucous membranes, ruptured blood vessels and trauma. Vigorous nose blowing or nose picking can sometimes induce a nosebleed. More serious chronic conditions, such as high blood pressure, arteriosclerosis, and bleeding diseases like hemophilia, may be involved.

Symptoms

Blood or blood tinged mucus either drips or is blown from the nose. Clots may form in the nose. Be careful if you remove these clots, or the nose may begin bleeding again.

Complications

Low blood volume and anemia may occur if the nosebleed will not stop and blood loss is extreme. If a nosebleed will not stop readily with direct pressure and homeopathic medicines, seek medical attention to find the source of the nosebleed.

Finding the Homeopathic Medicine

- For a nosebleed following an injury or trauma, give Arnica.
- For a bloody nose with a bright red face and a high fever, give Belladonna.
- If a child with a nosebleed has very pale cheeks, look at Ferrum phosphoricum.
- If the blood is dark, consider Hamamelis.
- For left sided nosebleeds with dark blood in a talkative person, consider Lachesis.
- If the person with the nosebleed asks for cold or carbonated drinks, look at Phosphorus.

Self Care and Home Remedies

- Apply direct pressure by squeezing the sides of the nose shut with thumb and forefinger for five to ten minutes while breathing through the mouth.
- Put a small piece of ice under the upper lip beneath the nose, or apply pressure to the point just under the nose on the upper lip.
- Apply a cold compress to the nose.

6

RESPIRATORY TRACT DISORDERS

Flu

Flu, or influenza is an acute illness caused by the body's response to viral infection by influenza viruses, types A, B, or C. It often comes in the form of epidemics in the winter.

Symptoms

People with the flu complain of headache, fever and chills, aching muscles and joints, fatigue, sore throat, and cough. There is less nasal secretion and more fatigue than with the common cold. Flu sufferers often feel "wiped out," and just want to stay in bed. Some influenza has a gastrointestinal component with nausea, vomiting and diarrhea.

Complications

Conventional medicine has no effective treatment for the flu. Babies and the elderly sometimes succumb to the flu if it is very severe or complicated by secondary bacterial infections, particularly pneumonia.

Finding the Homeopathic Medicine

- If the flu is just starting and there are no definite symptoms yet, choose Ferrum Phosphoricum.
- Oscillococcinum is available over the counter in many

pharmacies, health food stores, and supermarkets, and is our first choice at this stage unless high fever and red cheeks are prominent symptoms.

- After symptoms have developed, consider Bryonia if all the symptoms are made worse by movement and the person is very irritable and thirsty.
- Think about Gelsemium if the person is dizzy, drowsy, droopy, and dull, feels totally exhausted, and is not thirsty.
- Consider Eupatorium if the person feels deep aching in the bones and muscles and feels like his bones are broken.
- Give Rhus toxicodendron when stiffness is the main symptom, and it is made worse by cold damp weather or exertion, and better by stretching or moving around for a while.

Self Care and Home Remedies

- Rest.
- Drink plenty of fluids.
- If it is an upper respiratory flu, follow suggestions for Common Cold, Coughs, Bronchitis, and Fever.

Common Cold

The common cold is a viral infection associated with a large number of viruses that infect the nose, throat, and lungs.

Symptoms

Sore throat and stuffy nose, with a watery nasal discharge at first, then becoming thicker and colored. A low grade fever and headaches are common. A loose or dry, hacking cough often occurs as the cold "goes into the chest," and may persist for up to several weeks.

Complications

Colds may be complicated by bacterial infections leading to sinusitis and ear infections, and may progress to bronchitis or infrequently pneumonia.

Finding the Homeopathic Medicine

- Duing the first twenty four hours of a cold with a high fever, choose between Aconite, Belladonna, and Ferrum phosphoricum.
- If the symptoms fit Belladonna but it doesn't help use Ferrum phosphoricum.
- Allium cepa is the most common medicine for colds in which the eyes and nose run or drip like a faucet.
- Give Kali bichromicum if the main symptom is pressing pain in the sinuses and root of nose. The discharge will usually be thick, greenish-yellow, and stringy.
- If the symptoms come on after overwork or anger, and if the person is very impatient and irritable, look at Nux vomica.
- Pulsatilla is good for a ripe cold with thick yellow green discharge, changeable moods, and a whiny, clingy disposition.
- Give Arsenicum album for a cold with a watery, irritating nasal discharge in a chilly restless person who seems anxious and needy.
- People who need Mercurius are sensitive to both heat and cold, with yellow green mucus and bad breath.

Self Care and Home Remedies

- Drink two to four cups of hot ginger tea. Boil three slices of fresh ginger in two cups of water for fifteen minutes.

- Avoid dairy products, wheat, bananas and oatmeal because they increase mucus production.
- Vitamin C(500 mg every two hours, up to 3000mg per day) in the first stage of the cold.
- Beta-carotene: 50,000 IU per day
- Zinc: 30 mg per day.
- Zinc lozenges if there is a sore throat.
- Garlic capsules, two every four hours.
- Nasal wash with one-fourth teaspoon salt to one cup warm water once or twice a day. For the nasal wash, snuff a small amount of salt water from a cupped hand into the nostrils. Tilt your head back closing the throat, let the water drain into your mouth and spit it out.

Cough And Bronchitis

Acute bronchitis is an inflammation of the bronchial tubes of the lungs. It is often associated with a cold or upper respiratory infection, fever, sore throat, and a nasal discharge or postnasal drip. Although infection is the most common cause, it may also be caused by inhaling irritant substances, or it may be a complication of allergies and sinusitis. Bronchitis usually lasts three to five days, or up to several weeks.

Symptoms

Coughs may be dry or loose. The most common symptoms are a tickling feeling in the throat or chest, fits of uncontrollable coughing, excessive mucus, interrupted sleep due to the inability to lie down without coughing hoarseness and pain in the throat, chest or head.

Complications

Bronchitis may lead to pneumonia in serious cases. Patients with shortness of breath, weakness or exhaustion, persistent fever, and a thick yellow green, brown, or bloody mucus from the lungs should see a qualified homeopath or other medical practitioner immediately.

Finding the Homeopathic Medicine

If the cough is extremely loose and rattly, think first of Antimonium tartaricum, then of Ipecac and Pulsatilla.

- If the person feels parched and is worse from any movement, give Bryonia.
- For bronchitis with fits of coughing, look at Drosera, Hepar sulphuris, Spongia and Rumex.
- For dry, croupy coughs, think first of Spongia, Drosera and Hepar sulphuris.
- For coughs that come from a tickle in the pit of the throat look at Rumex.

Self Care and Home Remedies

- For a wet cough, drink three to four cups a day of hot ginger tea. Boil three slices of fresh ginger in two cups of water for fifteen minutes.
- Hot water with plenty of freshly squeezed lemon juice and a little honey helps cut mucus. Drink three to four cups a day.
- Gargle with warm salt water.
- Vitamin C: 500 mg every four hours.
- Beta carotene: 50,000 IU per day.
- Zinc: 30 mg per day.

- Drink licorice root tea, one cup three times a day, as an expectorant.
- Avoid dairy products, sweets, and heavy foods.

Sinusitis

Sinusitis is an inflammation of the sinuses associated with viral, bacterial, or fungal infections or allergies.

Symptoms

The most common symptom is mild to severe pain in the maxillary or frontal sinuses. There may also be pain in the face or teeth. There is generally nasal discharge or stuffiness and often a sinus headache. It is the deep sinus pain that usually differentiates sinusitis from the common cold.

Complications

A severe bacterial sinusitis left untreated could potentially cause a more serious systemic infection.

Finding the Homeopathic Medicine

- The first medicine to think of for sinusitis with pressing pain in the cheekbones and a thick, ropy nasal discharge is Kali bichromicum.
- If the sinusitis came after exposure to a draft, look first at Hepar sulphuris then at Nux vomica.
- If there are bad smelling odors in the nose and sinuses, think of Mercurius and Hepar sulphuris.
- If the sinusitis is much worse from going outdoors, think of Nux vomica and Hepar sulphuris.
- In a child with a sinus infection who is clingy, weepy, and moody, give Pulsatilla.

- If the sinusitis is much better from going outside, he probably needs Pulsatilla.

Self Care and Home Remedies

- Hot, moist packs applied to the sinuses can relieve congestion.
- Echinacea and goldenseal combination (two dropperfuls of tincture in water three times a day or six capsules a day) is useful to stimulate the immune system to fight infection.
- Give Vitamin A (25,000 IU per day) or betacarotene (50,000IU per day).
- Give Vitamin C (1000mg three times per day).
- Give Zinc (30mg per day).
- Nasal irrigation with one quarter teaspoon of salt in one cup of warm water can be very helpful. Plastic or porcelain neti pots are a particularly effective way to accomplish this.
- Hot, spicy food such as cayenne, black pepper, and horse radish can help clear the sinuses.
- Avoid dairy products sweets, and cold and carbonated drinks.
- Boil four slices of fresh ginger root in a quart of water for fifteen minutes and drink three to four cups a day.

7

MENTAL DISORDERS

Dizziness

Dizziness is a symptom more than an illness, but it is nonetheless quite annoying and can be debilitating. Dizziness may accompany fever, headache, and nausea in acute illnesses. It is also present with fainting, motion sickness and loss of balance.

Symptoms

Dizziness is often described as a loss of orientation, loss of balance and visual disturbance, often with a "lightheaded" feeling or a sensation of the room spinning. Nausea and vomiting often accompany the dizzy feeling.

Complications

- Dizziness may precede loss of consciousness and falling. It may be a symptom of more chronic, serious underlying problems with the endocrine or nervous system or the inner ear, such as hypothyroidism, multiple sclerosis, brain tumors, and meniere's disease. Dizziness may also come from breathing chemical fumes or from alcohol intoxication. Prolonged or recurrent dizziness should be diagnosed by a qualified homeopath or other qualified healthcare practitioner.

Finding the Homeopathic Medicine

- If the dizziness follows a fright or shock, give Aconite.

- Give Gelsemium for dizziness due to fright.
- When the dizziness is from motion or motion sickness, consider Bryonia or Cocculus first.
- Give Bryonia if the patient is very irritable, dry and thirsty and talks of business or wants to go home.
- If the dizziness is definitely from riding in a car or airplane or watching moving objects, give Cocculus.
- If the dizziness is associated with paralysis or weakness of the legs, you can try Conium first, but also see a homeopath as soon as possible.
- If the dizziness is associated with overall weakness, exhaustion, and dullness of mind, give Gelsemium.
- If the dizziness is worse during the menstrual period, when looking upward or from sitting down, in a weepy, clingy person who is worse in a warm, stuffy room, give Pulsatilla.

Self Care and Home Remedies

- Hold on to something to prevent falling.
- Do not drive or operate machinery while dizzy.
- Pick one point and look at it for orientation and balance.
- Sit or lie down; close your eyes.

Fainting

Fainting is a sudden brief loss of consciousness caused by a lowering of blood pressure to the brain. Faining may result from physical or emotional causes. Common causative factors are blood loss, dehydration, pain, fright, shock, becoming overheated, exhaustion, arrhythmias of the heart, overexertion, and hyperventilation.

Symptoms

Sudden loss of consciousness with collapse.

Complications

Fainting is usually brief and causes no harm other than the trauma from falling. Fainting may be a symptom of a more serious problem such as shock, head injury, heart attack, stroke or brain tumor. If pulse or breathing are absent, perform CPR (cardio-pulmonary resuscitation) immediately and have someone call for emergency medical assistance. If pulse and respiration are normal, but the person doesn't regain consciousness within a few minutes, seek immediate medical attention.

Finding the Homeopathic Medicine

- In cases of fainting due to an extreme fright, give Aconite first.
- For fainting following an accident or trauma, always give Arnica first.
- For fainting from hypothermia or drowning, give Carbo vegetabilis first, then consider Veratrum album.
- If the person has fainted follows excitement, give Coffea.
- For fainting from stage fright, Gelsemium is the best choice.
- Fainting from grief requires Ignatia.
- Hysterical fainting calls for Moschus.

Other Self - Care Suggestions

- Make sure the person has a clear airway.
- A cold washcloth on the forehead may help revive the person.

- Moisten the lips or tongue with a few drops of Bach Flower Essence Rescue Remedy; it will often work quickly to help revive the person.
- Make sure the person has fainted, rather than having suffered a serious injury or heart attack, before moving him.

Fever

Fever is a symptom, not a disease in itself. The body raises its temperature in order to fight infection when the immune system is in the process of responding to foreign invaders such as bacteria and viruses.

Symptoms

When your body temperature rises over 100°F, you have a fever. Fever is a beneficial reaction of the body to illness, and as such should be allowed to run its course unless it is very high. Chills often precede or accompany fever, and sweats occur when the fever is going down or "breaking." Fever may occur in the absence of infection, and in some cases it may be of unknown origin.

Complications

- Fever rarely goes above 105°F, but it may induce febrile seizures at that point. A high fever with a severely stiff neck may be caused by meningitis, a life-threatening disease that requires immediate medical attention. Homoeopathy is quite effective in dealing with the bacterial or viral infections that cause fever, even in cases in which antibiotics have failed. However, in serious infections with high fevers that do not respond to homoeopathy, medical attention should be sought.

Finding the Homeopathic Medicine

- Use Aconite or Belladonna for fevers that come on suddenly and violently.
- Fevers that need Aconite often start after a shock or fright or exposure to a cold dry wind.
- Belladonna is useful when the fever is high, the person's face is red, and the fever is accompanied by a throbbing headache.
- When the fever is intermittent or comes at the same time every day, consider China.
- Give Ferrum phosphoricum for fevers in the first stage of illness with few other symptoms than red cheeks.

Self Care and Home Remedies

- If fever is high, sponge your forehead, palms, soles and full body for half on hour. Then cover up the body.
- Drink plenty of water.
- Sage, basil or ginger tea may be of some help if cough accompanies fever.

Grief

Grief is an emotional reaction to loss and disappointment, such as the loss of a loved one, the breaking up of a relationship, or losing a job.

Symptoms

Grief is characterized by weeping, wailing, sobbing, sighing, withdrawal, and depression. Rational thinking is usually overcome by emotion during acute grief.

Complications

People who are grief stricken may become seriously depressed and even suicidal. If the person makes serious statements about suicide or makes any plans or attempts, emergency psychiatric intervention may be necessary.

Finding the Homeopathic Medicine

- Ignatia is the first medicine to think of in acute grief. If there is lots of sobbing and sighing and the person is hysterical give Ignatia.
- Natrum muriaticum is useful when the person is withdrawn, hides her tears from others, and desires salty food.
- Phosphoric acid should be given when the person is completely exhausted and apathetic after grief or hearing bad news.

Self Care and Home Remedies

- Confide your feelings to friends and family or a qualified therapist or spiritual counselor.
- Do not spend too much time alone.
- Let yourself cry until it passes on its own.
- Try not to dwell too much on the past, guilt, and regrets.
- Let the person or situation go, and move on with your life as soon as you are ready.
- Do something special for yourself to get your mind off your grief for a time.
- Do something to help someone else who needs it.

Insomnia

Insomnia is difficulty in falling asleep or staying asleep, to the point that it interferes with getting adequate rest. Insomnia may be caused by emotional distress, worry, nervous tension, too much thinking, pain, drugs, caffeine, overeating, or environments that are not conducive to sleeping.

Symptoms

People with insomnia either can't get to sleep, or they sleep too lightly and awaken too early or too frequently. They often feel tired in the morning upon waking, and do not dream normally.

Lack of sleep contributes to irritability, stress, poor performance at school or work, and a greater tendency to make mistakes or have accidents. People with chrnoic insomnia may become irritable or depressed.

Complications

An occasional lost night of sleep will not cause much difficulty, but chronic insomnia can take its toll on one's health. Sleep deprivation impacts the proper functioning of the immune system and decreases overall alertness and mental functioning.

Finding the Homeopathic Medicine

- If the person can't sleep following a terrifying experience, the medicine is Aconite.
- For insomnia that begins right after a financial crisis, give Arsenicum album.
- For someone who sits up in bed wide awake at 3:00 A.M., think of Coffea.
- Coffea and chamomilla can be helpful for sleeplessness due to hypersensitivity to pain.

- For inability to sleep because of anticipation or stage fright, Gelsemium fits best.
- If the insomnia began during a period of grieving after the death of a loved one, the best medicine is Ignatia.
- People who wake at 3:00 A.M. worrying about business often benefit from Nux vomica.

Self Care and Home Remedies

- Drink a cup of warm milk, containing the amino acid tryptophan, one half hour before bedtime.
- Equal parts of valerian root, skullcap, passionflower, and hops is a useful herbal sleep formula. Take thirty drops of tincture in warm water one half hour before bedtime or every two hours as needed.
- Take an hour of quiet time or relaxation without noise or entertainment before going to bed.
- Lie on the right side with arm outstretched to induce sleep more rapidly.
- Do alternate nostril breathing for five minutes at bedtime. Close the right nostril with your thumb pressed to the side of your nose. Inhale slowly through the left nostril. With your middle finger close the left nostril, release your thumb to open the right and exhale, Inhale through the right. Then close the right nostril and exhale through the left. Inhale slowly through the left and switch again, exhaling through the right. Continue for three to ten minutes.

Headache

Headache is simply pain in the head. It is more a symptom than a disease. Various kinds of headaches can occur, including tension headaches, migraine headaches and cluster headaches.

Symptoms

The pain of headaches may be localized, or may involve the entire head. It often begins in one place and extends to another. Many types of pain may occur, such as throbbing, bursting, aching, hammering, and so on. Migraine headaches are often one-sided; they arise from a circulatory problem, and involve visual disturbances, vomiting, and great sensitivity to noise, light, and jarring. Tension headaches often result from increased stress. Headaches in women may have a hormonal component.

Complications

Most headaches resolve on their own over time. Headaches that are very painful, persistent or recurrent may indicate a more serious underlying condition such as a brain tumor or brain aneurysm. Headaches may accompany serious acute illnesses, such as meningitis, strep throat, or other conditions with high fever. If you have very severe or persistent headaches, see a medical professional so that your condition may be properly diagnosed.

Finding the Homeopathic Medicine

- Headaches that are worse from the sun: Belladonna, Glonoine, Natrum Muriaticum, Sanguinaria.
- Lack of thirst with the headache: Belladonna, Gelsemium.
- Right sided headaches: Belladonna, Iris, Sanguinaria.
- Migraine headaches: Belladonna, Natrum muriaticum, Iris, Sanguinaria.
- Throbbing headaches: Belladonna, Glonoine, Sanguinaria.
- Sensitivitiy to light, noise, jarring: Belladonna, Sanguinaria.
- Very thirsty with the headache: Belladonna, Bryonia.

- Left sided headaches: Bryonia.
- Headaches made worse by motion: Bryonia.
- Bursting headaches: Bryonia, Glonoine.
- Dizzy, drowsy, droopy, and dull: Gelsemium.
- Migraine headaches with visual disturbances: Iris.
- Headaches from stomach problems: Iris, Sanguinaria.
- Headaches with a lot of vomiting: Iris, Sanguinaria.
- Migraines with herpes: Natrum muriaticum, Iris.
- Burning headaches like a hot wire or poker: Spigelia.

Self Care and Home Remedies

- Wrap a cold, wet cloth around your head or use an ice pack while you put your hands and feet in hot water.
- Lie down in a dark, quiet place.
- Play soft, soothing music.
- Do deep, slow breathing.
- Take a hot bath with one cup of Epsom salts.
- Massage your scalp and the trigger points on your neck and shoulders.
- Press deeply on the two points just below the flat bone at the back of the skull about two inches to either side of the center. Release when the pain goes away.

Shock

Shock is inadequate circulation of blood and oxygen to organs or tissues because of blood loss or dehydration, weak action of the heart, or dilation of the peripheral blood vessels.

Septic shock comes from bacterial infection. Anaphylactic shock comes from allergic reactions. Electric shock comes from exposure to live electric current of lightning.

Symptoms

The person is lethargic, sleepy, and confused. Hands and feet are clammy and pale or blue. The pulse and breathing are rapid and weak. In septic shock, fever and chills are usually present. Symptoms of anaphylactic shock include agitation, flushing, heart palpitations, numbness, itching, difficult breathing, hives, swelling, coughing, and sneezing followed by the general symptoms of shock. Electric shock may cause severe muscle contractions, loss of consciousness, heart palpitations or heart failure, and cessation of breathing; burns may also occur.

Complications

Shock is a medical emergency and can lead rapidly to death. Apply first aid measures immediately and call ambulance for emergency medical aid. Keep the person warm, raise his or her legs slightly, stop any blood loss with direct pressure if possible, check the person's airway and breathing, and give CPR (cardio pulmonary resuscitation) if necessary. Do not give anything by mouth that must be swallowed. (Homeopathic medicines may be dissolved in a small amount of water; a few drops on the tongue are sufficient for a dose.) Turn the head to allow the person to vomit if needed. Hospitalization is strongly recommended as intravenous fluids, drugs, or surgery may be needed depending on the cause of the shock.

Finding the Homeopathic Medicine

- Give Aconite for shock from fright, panic, or emotional causes.
- Arnica is very useful for shock from traumatic injuries and blood loss.

- Camphora is used for people who are extremely cold and worse from cold, but who paradoxically want cold drinks and to be uncovered.
- Carbo vegetabilisis the best medicine for acute shock when the person feels short of breath and wants to be fanned and cooled off.
- Carbolic acid is used in anaphylactic shock, especially from a bee sting.
- China is very good for shock from loss of bodily fluids, as in dehydration and blood loss.
- Veratrum album is good for shock after excessive vomiting, diarrhea, or blood loss.

8

MISCELLANEOUS DISORDERS

Abscesses

An abscess is an enclosed pocket in the tisue filled with pus, usually caused by the body's reaction to bacterial infection.

Symptoms

Abscesses are accompanied by heat, pain, swelling, redness, and tenderness over the site of the abscess. Fever may be present, but not always. Abscesses are difficult to heal without treatment.

Complications

Sometimes abscesses must be surgically drained in order to release the pus. If the abscess is severely painful, or if you observe any red streaks radiating from the area, get immediate medical attention.

Finding the Homeopathic Medicine

- Hepar sulphuris and Silica are the most common medicines for abscesses.
- For an abscess that is exquisitely sensitive to pain, cold, and touch, in a very irritable chilly person, give Hepar sulphuris.
- For an abscess from a foreign body give Silica unless the symptoms are particularly like Hepar sulphuris.

- For abscesses that are purplish or mottled, left-sided, and much better from discharging, in a talkative, intense person, give Lachesis.
- For abscesses that are very foul-smelling in a chilly, sweaty person with bad breath and a bad or metallic taste in the mouth, give Mercurius.

Self Care and Home Remedies

- If the abscess is draining, cover it with a gauze dressing and keep the area clean.
- Alternating hot (five minutes) and cold (one minute) wet compresses stimulates circulation and healing.
- Use massage teachniques of specifically promote drainage of the lymph system.
- A combination of echinacea and goldenseal (two dropperfuls of tincture in water three times a day or two capsules four times a day) can be useful to stimulate the immune system to fight infection.
- Apply Calendula tincture (diluted one part to three parts water) to the area once it has drained.
- Give betacartotene: 50,000 IU once a day.
- Give zinc: 30mg once a day.
- Give vitamin C: 1000mg two times a day.

Bleeding

Bleeding, or hemorrhage, is a flow of blood from the arteries, veins, or capillaries, occurring internally or through any of the natural openings of the body or from damage to the tissues or blood vessels. There are many causes of abnormal bleeding, ranging from wounds, trauma, and acute conditions, such as a nosebleed, to chronic conditions such as hemorrhoids, hemorrhagic disorders, or cancer.

Symptoms

Bleeding is characterized by a flow of blood, ranging in color from bright red to black, from anywhere in the body. The blood may spurt if it comes from an artery, or flow more passively if it originates in a vein. The most common symptoms of blood loss are weakness, fatigue, dizziness, a faint feeling, thirst, perspiration, and, later, changes in pulse and breathing. Anemia is confirmed through a complete blood count.

Complications

Extreme blood loss due to injury, postpartum hemorrhage (after childbirth), uncontrolled uterine bleeding due to other causes or undetected internal bleeding can result in anemia, dehydration, shock, or death. Get medical attention immediately if blood loss is severe.

Finding the Homeopathic Medicine

- The first medicine to give for bleeding resulting from injury or trauma is Arnica.
- For bleeding in which the person has bright red cheeks, consider Belladonna or Ferrum metallicum.
- For blood loss in a weak, pale, collapsed person, give China.
- If there is dark blood oozing from various parts of the body, give Crotalus horridus.
- For bleeding from the veins with a full feeling in the veins, the medicine is Hamamelis. If the bleeding is caused by a fall or overexertion and the blood is bright red, look at Millefolium.
- For a person who bleeds easily and the blood is fluid, bright red, and without clots, give phosphorus.

Self Care and Home Remedies

- Take whatever first-aid measures are necessary to stop the bleeding, including applying pressure directly to the injury with a clean cloth or by applying pressure to the pressure points above the injured area or by wrapping the injury with gauze or cloth.
- Apply Calendula tincture or a combination of Calendula and Hypericum tinctures directly to the bleeding area.
- Never apply topical Arnica preparations to open wounds because they can cause a rash.
- Dried cinnamon applied directly to the area can sometimes stop bleeding.
- Geranium, Trillium can all be taken internally for bleeding. Take one half teaspoon of tincture every one to two hours up to four times a day.

If weakness occurs from bleeding, take iron supplementation. The dosage depends on the form of iron, the degree of anemia and the cause and degree of bleeding.

Bruises

Bruises are caused by trauma that doesn't break the skin, resulting in blood leakage into the tissues.

Symptoms

Black and blue or purplish green discoloration under the skin with sore, aching, pain.

Complications

Discoloration may take a long time to go away, the area can remain tender.

Finding the Homeopathic Medicine

- Arnica is the first medicine to think for any bruise.
- Give Bellis perennis for bruises to the veins or from leakage from the veins after blood drawing or for ordinary bruises if Arnica fails.
- Give Ledum if the bruise is cold and feels better from cold.
- Give Ruta for bruises on the outer covering of bones (periosteum), such as on the shins.
- If the bruising tendency is chronic or recurrent, Phosphorus may work.
- Think of Sulphuric acid if Arnica doesn't work after injuries.

Self Care and Home Remedies

- Ice a bruise right away to keep more blood from leaking out into the tissues.
- Wrap an Ace bandage around the area, not too tightly, to support the area and control the extent of the bruise.
- After twelve hours, alternating hot and cold moist packs can help healing and remove discoloration.
- If a person is susceptible to bruising, bioflavonoids (1000mg per day) strengthen the veins.

Burns

Burns are caused by heat, electricity, radiation, hot water, or particular chemicals. The skin may be inflamed, blistered (second degree), or charred (third degree). The most common burns are sunburn and burns from fire or touching something hot.

Symptoms

- First degree: redness, heat, swelling, and pain.
- Second degree: all of the above plus blistering and oozing.
- Third-degree: significant charring of tissues.

Complications

Burns can be serious, even fatal, depending on the extent of the body that is burned and the degree of the burn. Any extensive burn–even first degree–should receive medical attention. First degree burns will heal without extensive treatment in most cases. Palliative treatment will help relieve pain and inflammation. Second and third degree burns may cause scarring and infection. Third-degree burns can be life threatening if extensive and may require treatment in a hospital setting. Get medical attention immediately for a third degree burn.

Chemicals will continue to burn the skin as long as they are present; wash them off immediately with lots of water. Get medical attention for serious electrical burns.

Finding the Homeopathic Medicine

- The first medicine to consider in most burns is Cantharis.
- For scalds, either give Cantharis first, then Urtica urens if there is not improvement within thirty minutes, or, if the other symptoms fit Urtica urens, give it first.
- For chemical burns, the after effects of old burns or burns that are slow to heal give Causticum.
- For electrical burns, give phosphorus.

Self Care and Home Remedies

- Soak the burned part in cold water or ice water, or apply cold wet compresses to relieve pain and inflammation.

Calendula or Hypericum tincture may be added to the water as described next.

- Apply Calendula spray, gel or tincture , diluted one part tincture to three parts water. Dilute more if the tinctue hurts to apply. Hypericum tincture may be used, diluted 1:3 as well. On first degree burns, Calendula gel or solution may be applied. Calendula tincture, diluted one part Calendula to three parts water, can be very useful in first and second degree burns.

Chicken Pox

Chicken pox is an acute viral disease, usually in young children, associated with the varicella zoster virus, which also causes shingles. It is spread by infected droplets from the nose or throat.

Symptoms

A period of mild headche, fever, and general discomfort followed by numerous fluid-filled sores, which crust over. Once crusts form, the contagious period is over. Normally once a person has chicken pox he will never get it again.

Complications

Chicken pox is very contagious and may cause scarring. The sores may become infected. Do not give aspirin to a child with chicken pox, because they may get Reye's syndrome–a type of brain and liver illness characterized by nausea and vomiting and a sudden change in mental functioning with lethargy, loss of memory, and disorientation, leading to coma.

Finding the Homeopathic Medicine

- The most common medicine for a very itchy chicken pox is Rhus toxicodendron.

- If the sores ooze a honey like discharge and scab over, and the tongue is coated white, think of Antimonium crudum.
- If the main symptom is a loose, rattling cough, take a look at Antimonium tartaricum.
- For out-of the ordinary fussiness in a child who doesn't want to be touched or looked at, consider Croton tiglium, especially if the skin feels very tight.
- If the child is very clingy, weepy, and thirstless, look at Pulsatilla.

Self Care and Home Remedies.

- Oatmeal bath: use Aveno (avoid the type that contains camphor) or place one cup of finely blended dry oatmeal in the bath to soothe the itching.
- To treat infected sores, apply a few drops of one part Calendula tincture diluted with three parts water and cover with bandages or gauze.

Cuts, Scrapes, and Puncture Wounds

A wound is caused by a sharp object piercing the skin. It may be a cut (laceration or incision), a puncture wound, or a scrape (abrasion).

Symptoms

Tissue damage, bleeding, bruising, inflammation, swelling, and pain are the most prominent symptoms of wounds. The seriousness of the wound depends on the amount of damage to underlying organs and tissues.

Complications

Superficial wounds are not serious, and usually heal rapidly on their own if they are kept clean free of infection. Deep cuts may need stitches. If cuts or puncture wounds are deep, damage to organs, muscles, nerves and bones needs to be assessed immediately by a qualified medical practitioner. A sserious wound, such as a knife or gunshot wound, may be life threatening.

Puncture wounds carry the risk of tetanus within two days to two months after a wound has been infected. Deep or dirty puncture wounds should have dirt and dead tissue removed by a qualified medical practitioner to help prevent tetanus. Early signs of tetanus include jaw stiffness, difficulty swallowing and stiffness of the neck, arms, or legs after a wound. More advanced tetanus includes the inability to open the jaw (lockjaw), a fixed smile, and raised eyebrows, as well as spasms in the neck, back and abdomen. Tetanus may be fatal if untreated. If the person has not had a tetanus immunization or booster in the last five years, a tetanus inoculation should be given immediately following the injury. A dose of homeopathic Ledum may be given immediately as well.

Finding the Homeopathic Medicine

- The first medicines to consider for puncture wounds are Ledum and Hypericum.
- If the affected part is cold and cold to the touch, give Ledum.
- If there is numbness or shooting pains, use Hypericum.
- If there is bruising or bleeding, give Arnica.

Self Care and Home Remedies

- For serious wounds: Apply direct pressure to stop bleeding. Get medical attention immediately.
- For minor wounds: Apply direct pressure to stop bleeding. Clean the wound with soap and water.

- Apply Calendula gel, cream, or spray (for abrasions), or tincture, diluted one part tincture to three parts water. Dilute more if the tincture hurts when applied. Calendula prevents and heals infections. Hypericum tincture may be used, diluted one to three parts as well, especially for infected cuts or scrapes. Use the tinctures several times a day until there is definite healing, then once a day until healing is complete.
- Cover the wound with a bandage or gauze dressing.
- Change the dressing as needed.
- For minor puncture wounds: Clean the wound with soap and water.
- Let the wound bleed freely to flush out diret or debris unless bleeding is severe.
- For severe bleeding: Apply direct pressure on the wound. Soak puncture wounds in warm water several times a day to remove more debris.
- Apply full strength or diluted Calendula tincture to promote healing.
- For general wound healing: Vitamin C (500 mg four times a day).
- Zinc (30mg per day).
- Beta-carotene (50,000 IU per day).

Insect Bites and Stings

Everyone has had the experience of a bee sting or an insect bite. It is usually just annoying, painful, or inconvenient, putting a damper on a perfect outing or picnic. Sometimes it can cause a severe allergic reaction or anaphylactic shock.

Symptoms

Redness, swelling and itching occur after the bite, sometimes with burning or stinging pain. Hives, difficult breathing, and shock may occur with severe anaphylactic reactions. Signs of anaphylactic shock are paleness, perspiration, confusion or unconsciousness, rapid pulse and shallow, irregular breathing.

Complications

Occasionally the person who is bitten or stung can have a severe allergic or anaphylactic reaction, which can be life threatening. This may occur from a second bite or sting when there was not much reaction to the first one . Get medical attention immediately if the bite is from a poisonous insect or spider, or if there is difficutly in breathing, severe swelling, or loss of consciousness. Consult a physician if you think the person may have been exposed to Lyme disease; a red circle resembling a target around the site of a deer tick bite is one early symptom. Antibiotics may be necessary to avoid later complications of heart and muscle or joint disease.

Finding the Homeopathic Medicine

- The first medicine to give if there is swelling is Apis.
- For bee stings, give Apis.
- For bites with terrific itching, consider Caladium.
- In the case of anaphylactic shock, call ambulance and give Carbolic acid or Apis.
- For most insect bites, first try Ledum.
- For wasp stings, Vespa is the first choice. Use Apis if Vespa is not available.

Self Care and Home Remedies

- Remove the stinger with a flicking motion using a fingernail or a sterilized needle. Pulling it straight out may release additional venom.
- Apply an ice pack or a cold, moist pack to reduce swelling and circulation, and to prevent the spread of the venom.
- Clense the area with soap and water.
- Calendula (Marigold flower) cream can ease itching and irritation.

Measles

Measles is a viral disease that affects children and adults who do not have active immunity. It is highly contagious and is spread by airborne droplets from an infected person before the rash apears and during the first few days of the disease.

Symptoms

Fever (up to 104°F), runny nose, sore throat, cough, sensitivity to light, and an extensive pink to brownish pink, irregular, itchy rash starting around the ears, face, and neck which then lightens up as it spreads to the trunk and limbs as the fever decreases. Koplik spots, which appear only in measles, look like tiny grains of sand with a red ring and are usually seen opposite the first and second upper molars on the inside of the cheek.

Complications

Secondary infections with streptococci and other bacteria may occur causing pneumonia, ear infections, and other infections. In one out of a thousand children, measles can cause encephalitis with fever, convulsions, and coma.

Finding the Homeopathic Medicine

- Give Aconite if the symptoms come on suddenly and violently with a high fever, especially after a fright or exposure to cold dry wind.
- Euphrasia is used for measles when there is a lot of sensitivity to light and a discharge from the eyes.
- Gelsemium is the medicine when measles comes on more slowly and the child is dizzy, drowsy, droopy and dull with a fever and headache in the back of the head.
- Pulsatilla is used in the later stages of measles when thick yellow green discharge and a low fever are present and the rash is beginning to fade.
- Sulphur is used when the rash is late to develop, and is purplish or dusky and the itching is made worse by heat and bathing.

Self Care and Home Remedies

- Bed rest in a darkened room.
- Drink plenty of fluids.
- Eat a light diet, depending on appeite.
- Vitamin C: 250 mg twice a day for young children, 500mg two times a day for adults.
- Keep sores clean and avoid scratching them.
- Apply cold compresses to the sores.

Motion Sickness

Motion sickness, also known as sea, air, or car sickness, is a complex of symptoms caused by stimulation of the balance mechanism in the inner ear by repeated motion. Disorientation, without being able to see a fixed horizon during motion, can induce motion sickness. It can be compounded by emotional stress.

Symptoms

Nausea and vomiting are the primary symptoms. Salivation, sweating, paleness, and hyperventilation are also common. Mental confusion can also be present.

Complications

Dehydration and lack of eating can produce problems if the motion sickness is prolonged.

Finding the Homeopathic Medicine

- Cocculus is the most common medicine for motion sickness.
- Petroleum is good for the combination of motion sickness and skin problems.
- Sepia is useful for motion sickness that is complicated by hormonal problems or relieved by vigorous exercise.
- Tabacum should be used when motion sickness is extemely severe.

Self Care and Home Remedies

- Try to sit in the place in the vehicle where there is the least motion. Stare at a fixed point for orientation, not at anything that is moving.
- Lying down or reclining may help.
- Look above the horizon at a forty five degree angle.
- Get some fresh air.
- Eat small amounts of food frequently.
- Eat Saltime crackers to help relieve the nausea.
- Eat bland foods such as broth, rice, and pasta.
- Tea and toast are usually well tolerated.

- Sip ginger root tea to help relieve nausea.
- Stimulate stomach, an acupressure point in the soft place below the knee and to the outside of the leg where the tibia and fibula bones meet. Use firm rotary pressure on the spot for a few seconds. Repeat when needed.

Suntroke, Heatstroke and Heat Exhaustian

These are conditions resulting from oversensitivity or prolonged exposure to the heat or the sun.

Symptoms

Heatstroke, also called sunstroke, is a reaction to exposure to the sun which often begins with a headache, dizziness, and fatigue leading to heat, flushig, and dryness of the skin. Perspiration is usually, but not always, decreased. The pulse rate increases quickly, sometimes up to 180 beats per minute, and breathing rate often increases also. The person can become disoriented and unconscious, as well as having seizures. Body temperature can shoot up very quickly to 104°F or even 106°F.

Heat exhaustion, which is less severe, is characterized by gradual weakness, nausea, profuse perspiration, anxiety, and fainting. The skin is generally pale and clammy. The pulse is weak and the blood pressure is low. Notice that the primary differences between the two are perspiration and the pulse.

Complications

In heatstroke, collapse of the heart can lead to permanent brain damage or death. Heat exhaustion is usually temporary and rarely has complications. If the body temperature is rising rapidly and the person has the symptoms of heatstroke/sunstroke, seek emergency medical attention.

Finding the Homeopathic Medicine

- Belladonna and Glonoine have very similar indications for this condition. Unless the main complaint is a bursting or exploding sensation in the head, give Belladonna first.
- If there is no improvement within fifteen minutes, or if there are other clear symptoms that point to Glonoine, give Glonoine.

Self Care and Home Remedies

For heatstroke: Take immediate measures to cool yourself by taking a cold shower or bath, or wrapping yourself in cold towels or ice.

For heat exhaustion: lie with the head down. Replace fluids and salt.

Hay Fever

Hay fever, or acute allergic rhinitis, is a reaction to pollens from grasses, trees, and flowers. Bouts of hay fever often occur annually when pollens are released, generally in the spring, summer, or fall.

Symptoms

Runny nose with clear watery discharge, sneezing and itchy eyes, nose, and mouth are the common symptoms. Headache and irritability often accompany hay fever. People who have it often feel miserable. Many hay fever sufferers also have allergies at other times of the year.

Finding the Homeopathic Medicine

- The most common medicine for hay fever with watery eyes, watery nasal discharge and sneezing is Allium cepa.

- If there is an irritating discharge from the nose and a bland discharge from the eyes, consider Allium cepa.
- If itching of the nose and palate is the primary symptom, give Arundo or Wyethia.
- When eye symptoms, especially watering are the most significant symptoms, give Euphrasia.
- When the eye discharge is irritating but the nasal discharge is bland, give Euphrasia.
- When the discharge is like egg white and the person has cold sores or canker sores, a headache, and perhaps a recent disappointment, rejection, or grief, Natrum muriaticum is the medicine.
- If sneezing is the most prominent symptom, strongly consider Sabadilla.

Self Care and Home Remedies

- Use an indoor air purifier to remove pollens from the air.
- Vaccum your living and work areas more often during hay fever season.
- Bioflavonoids can be helpful.
- Take 500 mg of Vitamin C twice a day.

Fever

Fever is a symptom, not a disease in itself. The body raises its temperature in order to fight infection when the immune system is in the process of responding to foreign invaders such as bacteria and viruses.

Symptoms

When your body temperature rises over 100°F, you have a fever. Fever is a beneficial reaction of the body to illness, and as such should be allowed to run its course unless it is very high. Chills often precede or accompany fever, and sweats occurwhen the fever is going down or "breaking." Fever may occur in the absence of infection, and in some cases it may be of unknown origin.

Complications

- Fever rarely goes above 105°F, but it may induce febrile seizures at that point. A high fever with a severely stiff neck may be caused by meningitis, a life-threatening disease that requires immediate medical attention. Homoeopathy is quite effective in dealing with the bacterial or viral infections that cause fever, even in cases in which antibiotics have failed. However, in serious infections with high fevers that do not respond to homoeopathy, medical attention should be sought.

Finding the Homeopathic Medicine

- Use Aconite or Belladonna for fevers that come on suddenly and violently.
- Fevers that need Aconite often start after a shock or fright or exposure to a cold dry wind.
- Belladonna is useful when the fever is high, the person's face is red, and the fever is accompanied by a throbbing headache.
- When the fever is intermittent or comes at the same time every day, consider China.
- Give Ferrum phosphoricum for fevers in the first stage of illness with few other symptoms than red cheeks.

Self Care and Home Remedies

- If fever is high, sponge you forehead, palms, soles and may be complete body for half on hour. Then cover up the body.
- Drink plenty of water.
- Sage, basil or ginger tea may be of some help if cough accompanies fever.

9

HOMOEOPATHIC MATERIA MEDICA

[Remedies And Their Indications]

Here is a brief summary of homoeopathic remedies; which are necessary to keep in house.

ACONITUM NAPELLUS (ACONITE)

- Ailments from fright; sudden onset and intense symptoms.
- Anxiety and restlessness with any complaint.
- Intolerant of pain, fears will not recover.
- Pains followed by numbness and tingling.
- Faintness or dizziness on rising.
- Common cold, first stages only.
- Fevers; sudden onset; hot, dry skin; often one cheek red, the other pale.
- Thirst for large quantities of water, unquenchable.
- Painful, red, hot, scanty urination, with anxiety.
- Croup; when child wakes frightened from sleep with dry, hoarse, croupy cough. Usually the only remedy needed.
- Eyes; relieves pain and aids healing in injuries such as a scratch on the eyeball, or pain from a foreign body in the eye.
- Bursting, throbbing headache; sensation as if band around head.

WORSE FROM

Evening and night, lying on affected side, warm room, music, tobacco smoke, dry, cold winds.

BETTER FROM

Open air.

ALLIUM CEPA

- Colds in damp, cold weather. Onset with sneezing. Streaming eyes and nose. Nasal discharge acrid, making upper lip and nose sore. Discharge from eyes in bland.
- Nose stuffed.
- Only one nostril dripping.
- Hoarseness, beginning laryngitis.
- Coughs from inhaling cold air. Grasps throat when coughing; feels as if cough would split or tear it.
- Headache, mostly in forehead.
- Neuralgic pains.
- Indicated in colicky babies with pains in the abdomen.
- Symptoms begin on the left side and extend toward the right.

WORSE FROM

Evening, warm room.

BETTER FROM

Open air, cold room.

ANTIMONIUM TARTARICUM (ANTIM. TART.)

- Cough; rattling of mucus in chest, but nothing comes up.

- Wheezing. Difficult breathing as if drowning in own secretions.
- Face is cold, blue, pale, covered with cold sweat.
- Great sleepiness.

WORSE FROM

Damp, cold weather, evening, warmth, all sour foods, milk.

BETTER FROM

Cold, open room, sitting up, belching, spitting.

APIS MELLIFICA (APIS)

- Bee stings and insect bites with swelling, itching, and redness.
- Hives.
- Pains are stinging and burning
- Puffy swellings may be around the face, eyelids, eyes, mouth, or in throat.
- Breathing difficult.
- Thirstless.
- Scanty urine.

WORSE FROM

Heat, touch, bed is intolerable, pressure, right side, late afternoon, after sleeping, closed, heated room.

BETTER FROM

Cold applications, motion, open air, uncovering.

ARNICA MONTANA (ARNICA)

- Bruising injuries to soft tissues.
- Injuries from blows, falls, or blunt objects.

- Shock from injury.
- Concussion of the brain.
- Eye injuries, black eye.
- Bleeding caused by injury.
- Promotes healing.
- Relieves soreness and bruised feeling following childbirth, illnesses, fractures, and surgery.
- Soreness after tooth extraction or dental surgery.
- Soreness of muscles from overexertion.
- Sprains of joints, "tennis elbow."
- Helpful even in old injuries.
- Denies he or she is ill or that there is anything wrong.
- Everything on which patient lies seems too hard.
- Fear of being touched or of anyone's coming near.

WORSE FROM

Light touch, heat, rest.

BETTER FROM

Lying down, with head low.

ARSENICUM ALBUM (ARSENICUM)

- Anxious, restless, fearful, irritable.
- Weak and exhausted.
- Desires air but is sensitive to the cold.
- Later stages of head cold, with sneezing; red nose and eyes; and profuse, watery discharge.
- Asthma worse after midnight; fears suffocation while lying down.

- Burning pains, better from heat.
- Sleepiness but unable to sleep; restlessness.
- Thirsty for small drinks often.
- Food poisoning.
- Vomiting with or without offensive diarrhea after eating or drinking, followed by great weakness.

WORSE FROM

Right side, after midnight, sight or smell of food, cold, cold drinks and food.

BETTER FROM

Warmth, head elevated, hot drinks.

BELLADONNA

- Restless, red, and hot.
- Cold, flu, sore throat, cough, fever, headache, earache.
- Earaches, especially the right ear, after getting the head cold or wet. Sudden onset.
- Fever, especially in children. Pupils dilated, eyes bright.
- Sudden and violent onset.
- Skin dry and hot to the touch.
- Eyes red, sensitive to the light, pupils dilated.
- Throbbing, congestive headaches.
- Sleepy but can't sleep. Restless sleep with muscular twitching.
- Teething problems.
- Sunstroke with pounding pulse.
- Throbbing pains, worse from motion or jarring.
- Vomiting from fright or nervousness.

WORSE FROM

Motion, noise, jarring, light, lying down

BETTER FROM

Standing or sitting erect

BRYONIA ALBA (BRYONIA)

- Conditions with fever.
- Dry, hard, spasmodic cough with stitches in the chest; must press hand to sternum. Cough worse at night, after eating and drinking, taking a deep breath, and when entering a warm room.
- Headaches; head feels as if it would burst. Pain sharp from slightest cough. Thirsty, but drinking makes headache worse.
- Wants to be quiet and left alone. Irritable. Wants things, which are refused when offered.
- Pale.
- Feverish.
- Thirsty for large amounts of cold drinks at long intervals.
- Constipated; stools large, dry, and hard.
- Colic, vomiting from rich or fatty foods.
- Rheumatism with red, swollen, hot, shiny joints. Motion, touch and pressure aggravate the pain.
- Symptoms develop slowly, usually worse on right side.

WORSE FROM

Motion, light touch, warmth, exertion, eating.

BETTER FROM

Rest, firm pressure, lying on painful side, because it prevents motion, cold.

CALCAREA PHOSPHORICA (CALC. PHOS.)

- Pains in joints and bones, "growing pains."
- Delayed or difficult teething in children, rapid decay of teeth.
- Delayed closure of fontanellies in top of child's head.
- Debility with anemia, sweaty scalp.
- Colic whenever child eats, feeble digestion.
- Easy vomiting in children.
- Craving for ham, bacon, smoked or salted meats.
- Promotes milk flow for breastfeeding mothers, when other symptoms agree.
- Fractures where bones do not unite or are slow to do so.
- Sensations of numbness and crawling.

WORSE FROM

Damp, cold, changeable weather, mental exertion.

BETTER FROM

Summer, warm, dry weather.

CANTHARIS

- Cystitis; frequent burning, painful urination.
- Intolerable constant urge to urinate.
- Burns and scalds with rawness and smarting, relieved by cold applications.
- Cantharis aids healing and takes away the burning sensation.
- Burning sensation in esophagus and stomach.
- Burning in soles of feet at night.
- Unquenchable thirst with aversion to all fluids.
- Bad effects of drinking coffee.

WORSE FROM

Drinking coffee and cold water, touch, urinating.

BETTER FROM

Gentle massage.

CARBO VEGETABILIS (CARBO VEG.)

- Weakness; desire for fresh, cold air.
- Sudden collapse from any cause.
- Breath cold.
- Limbs cold, bluish skin, sweat cold and clammy.
- External or internal bleeding with steady oozing.
- Internal burnings and external coldness.
- Aversion to milk and meat.
- All foods disagree, turn to gas, especially fats. Gas worse lying down.
- Burning in the stomach with sour belching, flatulence, regurgitation of food and heartburn.
- Rattling cough with itching in the throat. Spasmodic cough with gagging, choking and vomiting of mucus.
- Hoarseness, worse evenings.
- Has never fully recovered from the effects of some previous illness.

WORSE FROM

Evening, warm, moist weather, lying down, fat foods, wine, coffee, milk.

BETTER FROM

Fanning, cold, belching.

CHAMOMILLA

- Intolerance of pain; fainting and sweating from severe pain.
- Sensitive, peevish, irritable children. Child ask for things, wants to be carried.
- Painful teething with or without fever. Greenish diarrhea during teething.
- Colic; painful, draws legs up.
- One cheek hot, the other pale and cold.
- Toothache better from cold. Worse from warm drinks and at night.
- Earache with severe pain. Ears feel stopped.
- Thirsty.

WORSE FROM

Heat, open air, wind, night.

BETTER FROM

Being carried, warm, wet weather.

FERUM PHOSPHORICUM (FERRUM PHOS.)

Early stages of all inflammatory problems, including head colds, earache, cough, pneumonia, bronchitis, pleurisy and rheumatism. Fever with gradual onset. Pale complexion with red cheeks. Soft and rapid pulse. Hard, dry, ticking cough, with painful chest and hoarseness. Throbbing headache that is better from cold applications. Symptoms usually worse on right side.

WORSE FROM

At night, motion.

BETTER FROM

Cold applicatioins, 4 to 6 A.M., touch.

GELSEMIUM SEMPERVIRENS (GELSEMIUM)

- Summer colds with mild fever. Watery discharge from nose with much sneezing. Dry cough with sore throat.
- Influneza.
- Tiredness and aching of whole body. Limbs, head, eyelids feel heavy.
- Chilled with chills up and down back.
- Headache as if band around head. Scalp sore to the touch.
- Sore throat with red tonsils. Difflcult swallowing.
- Pain shoots from throat to ear. lack of thist.
- Dizziness, drowsiness, trembling and dullness.
- Bad effect of sun or hot weather.
- Symptoms develop several days after exposure.
- Nervousness, apprehension, anxiety prior to dental work or surgery.

WORSE FROM

Damp weather, emotion, anticipation, any effort to think, thinking or one's ailments, tobacco smoking.

BETTER FROM

Bending forward, open air, continued motion, increased urination, stimulants.

HEPAR SULPHURIS CALCAREUM (HEPAR SULPH.)

- Irritable. Chilly.
- Great sensitivity mentally and physically.
- Sensitive to cold, cold air, drafts. Feels as if wind is blowing on some part.

- Faints from slight pain.
- Cold sores, abscesses, boils, infected ears.
- Cold begins with irritation in throat.
- Sore, ulcerated nose. Sneezes when goes into cold, dry wind, nose runs; later there is a thick, offensive discharge.
- Sore throat with splinter sensation. Pain extends to ears when swallowing.
- Hoarseness with loss of voice.
- Dry, hoarse cough. Worse whenever any part of body becomes uncovered.
- Croup with loose, rattling cough.
- This remedy also helps to localize infection.

WORSE FROM

Dry, cold air, touch, lying on painful side, slightest draft, cool air.

BETTER FROM

Wet weather, warmth, wrapping head up, eating.

HYPERICUM PERFOLIATUM (HYPERICUM)

- Helpful in injuries to nerves.
- Puncture wounds, nails, bites, splinters.
- Smashed fingertips, nails, or toes.
- Pain shoots upward from the wound, especially up the limbs, or, in spinal injury, up and down the spine.
- Severe concussions of the spine and the brain. Injury to the tailbone or coccyx.
- Bee stings, if pains shoot upward.
- Dental surgery, including root canal work or tooth extraction.

- Eye injury.
- Relieves pain after operations.
- Speeds healing of jagged cuts.
- Painful burns, as a lotion: ½ teaspoon to 1 cup water.

WORSE FROM

Dampness, fog, touch, cold.

BETTER FROM

Bending head back.

IGNATIA AMARA (IGNATIA)

- Emotional strain.
- Mental stress.
- Bad effects of grief, worry, shock and disappointment.
- Hysteria.
- Sad, sighing, moody, changeable.
- Hiccough and hysterical vomiting.
- Insomnia.
- Headache as if nails were driven out through the side. Often follows anger or grief. Worse from stooping.
- Intolerance of tobacco.

WORSE FROM

Morning, emotions, tobacco smoke, coffee, brandy, strong odors.

BETTER FROM

Lying on the painful side, warmth, walking, hard pressure.

IPECACUANHA (IPECAC)

- Persistent nausea and vomiting, with a clean tongue.
- Nausea not relieved by vomiting.

- Lack of thirst.
- Asthma attacks.
- Cough incessant and violent with every breath.
- Nosebleed.
- Gushing of bright, red blood.
- Gasping for air.
- Pale, cold sweat.
- Pulse weak.

WORSE FROM

Lying down, slightest motion, dry weather.

LEDUM PALUSTRE (LEDUM)

- Helpful for puncture wounds from sharp-pointed objects such as nails and splinters.
- Insect stings, especially mosquitoes.
- Animal bites and scratches.
- Black eye caused by a blow.
- Injured parts are cold and are relieved by cold applications.

WORSE FROM

Warm applications, heat of the bed, night.

BETTER FROM

Cold applications

MAGNESIA PHOSPHORICA (MAGNESIUM PHOS.)

- Intermittent, spasmodic pains and neuralgia.
- Colic with gas, better from gentle pressure and warmth.
- Colic with belching, which gives no relief.
- Frequent hiccoughs with heartburn.

- Cramping pains, in calves, writer's cramp, menstrual cramps if relieved by heat.
- Toothache relieved by heat.
- Symptoms usually worse on the right side.
- General muscular weakness.

WORSE FROM

Cold, touch, night.

BETTER FROM

Warmth, gentle pressure, bending double.

MERCURIUS VIVUS (MERCURIUS)

- Smarting, raw, sore throat. Tonsillitis.
- Swollen, inflamed neck glands.
- Abscessed ears, pus infection, boils.
- Profuse sweating with no relief. Offensive odor.
- Bad breath. Profuse, metallic-tasting saliva.
- Very thirsty, even though mouth is moist.
- Thick tongue with yellowish-whiter coating. Teeth leave an imprint on the tongue.
- Swollen gums with soreness about teeth.
- Painful diarrhea with a "never get done" feeling.
- Persistent urging to urinate with intensive burning.
- Extremely sensitive to heat and cold.
- Weak and trembling.

WORSE FROM

Night, warmth of bed, during perspiration, heat and cold, damp weather.

BETTER FROM

Being at rest.

NUX VOMICA (NUX)

- Irritable, impatient, hypersensitive to noise, touch, light, odors, etc.
- Nausea, vomiting; sour, bitter belching, especially after improper eating or overindulgence in food or drink. Worse in the morning and after eating.
- Chilly, sensitive to drafts.
- Bad effects of coffee, alcoholic beverages, tobacco, highly seasoned foods, loss of sleep or strong drugs.
- Constipation with frequent and ineffectual urging for stool.
- Headache in back of head or over eyes, as if nail is driven in. Dizziness.
- Colds from dry, cold weather.
- Nose stuffed, especially at night and in the open air. Nose drips during the day and in a warm room.
- Insomnia after mental strain, abuse of coffee, alcohol, tobacco. Wakes between 3 and 4 A.M., falls asleep at daybreak, unrefreshed on waking.

WORSE FROM

Early morning, mental exertion, anger, eating, dry weather, touch, spices, stimulants, narcotics, cold, open air.

BETTER FROM

Rest, evening, strong pressure, uninterrupted nap, warmth

PHOSPHORUS

- Anxious, fearful, weak.

- Profuse bleeding anywhere. Nosebleed from vigorous nose blowing. Bleeding gums.
- Hoarseness, loss of voice.
- Painful laryngitis, tight, heavy chest.
- Croupy, dry, rasping, tickling, tight cough, which is very exhausting. Worse from talking or breathing cold air.
- Burning pains in stomach, intestines, and between shoulder blades.
- Thirst for ice-cold drinks, which are vomited as soon as they become warm in the stomach.
- Nausea.
- Symptoms are worse on the left side.
- Appears to be well despite high temperature.
- Sweats at night.

WORSE FROM

Evening, lying on left or painful side, physical or mental exertion, thunderstorms, change of weather, getting wet in hot weather, warm food or drink, touch

BETTER FROM

Open air, sleep, rubbing, cold food or drink.

PULSATILLA NIGRICANS (PULSATILLA)

- Sensitive, weepy, desires attention and sympathy.
- Changeable symptoms.
- Craves open air, sensitive to heat.
- Dryness of mouth with lack of thirst.
- Stomach upsets from rich foods. Aversion to fats.
- Fainting from hot stuffy atmosphere.

- Insomnia from recurring thought.
- "Ripe" head colds with profuse, thick, yellowish discharge. Eyelids stick together in the morning.
- Styes.
- Loose, rattling cough, worse on becoming heated and at night.
- Earache with thick yellow discharge. External ear swollen and red.
- Often indicated in allergies, as hayfever, asthma, eczema.
- Helpful in childhood diseases such as measless, mumps and chickenpox.
- To dry up mother's milk when no longer needed.
- Delayed menstrual period with painful, scanty flow.

WORSE FROM

Twilight, rich, fatty food, after eating, warm room, lying on left or painless side.

BETTER FROM

Motion, open air, cold food and drinks, though not thirsty, cold applications.

RUTA GRAVEOLENS (RUTA)

- Sprains (after *Arnica*), especially of tendons.
- Helps in sprains of knees, wrists, ankles.
- Injured, "bruised" bones, eyes, rectum, periosteum (the membrane surrounding the bone).
- Painful, bruised skin.
- Sciatica, worse lying down at night.
- Red, hot eyes, eyestrain followed by headache.

- Deep aching.
- "Dry socket" following dental extraction.

WORSE FROM

Being at rest, lying down, cold, wet weather, cold.

SPONGIA TOSTA (SPONGIA)

- Croup, colds and coughs beginning in the throat, which is sensitive to touch. Feeling as if there's a plug in the larynx.
- Wakes fearfully out of sleep with a sense of suffocation, loud cough, difficult breathing.
- Croupy cough, sounds like a saw driven through a board. Dry, barking, rasping cough.
- Dryness of all air passages.
- Hoarseness with soreness and burning.
- Exhaustion and heaviness of the body after slight exertion.
- Symptoms are similar to *Hepar sulph.* Symptoms except that the *Spongia* patient is warm while the *Hepar sulph.* Patient is chilly.

WORSE FROM

Before midnight, lying down, talking, swallowing, waking.

BETTER FROM

Lying with head low.

SULPHUR

- Dry, scaly, unhealthy skin, with itching and burning, offensive odor. Worse from scrathing and washing.
- Red orifices, lips, eyelids, anus.
- Burning heat of palms, top of head and especially soles of feet at night, uncovers feet, throws off bedcovers.

- Uncomfortable when standing.
- Dislike of water. Bathing makes patient feel worse.
- Hypoglycemic symptoms, sinking feeling in stomach an hour before lunch time.
- Thirsty, would rather drink than eat.
- Bitter taste in the morning.
- Painless diarrhea drives patient out of bed in early morning.
- Constipation with hard, dry, large stools, held back because of pain, helpful in anal fissures (cracks inside anus) burning.
- Sometimes helpful in failure to recover completely from acute ailments, as when colds, coughs, influenzas hang on too long.

WORSE FROM

Morning, night, washing, sleeping, rest, standing, warmth of bed, time to time, alcoholic stimulants.

BETTER FROM

Dry, warm weather, lying on right side.

VERATRUM ALBUM (VERATRUM ALB.)

- Nausea with violent vomiting and profuse diarrhea, clammy sweating and collapse.
- Cramping, watery diarrhea.
- Heat exhaustion.
- Sudden collapse with coldness, blueness, and weakness.
- Clammy sweat. Cold sweat on forehead.
- Pulse rapid and weak.
- Cramps in abdomen, legs, and calves.

WORSE FROM

Night, least motion, drinking, during stool, after fright.

BETTER FROM

Warmth, walking.

HOMEOPATAHIC TREATMNT ON THE BASIS Of WEEPING

- Weeps when he wants to walk in fever : Bryonia.
- Weeps all the night but sleeps durnig the day time. Jalapa.
- Grasps and catches hold of the rib due to fear of falling down and does not sleep: Borax
- Weeps profusely at the time of birth. Medorrh.
- Weeps as if frightened from seeing some horible object: Stramonium.
- Weeps due to colic or abdominal pain: Cuprum Met, Mag Phos.
- Weeps and afraid to breath: Belladonna.
- Weeps due to gripes for an hour after taking milkfeed: Nux Vomica.
- Is obstinate and demands odd things but quietens only when demanded and desired thing is given to him: Chamomilla.
- Weeps from 4 am to 9 pm. bores his feet into pubes, tenesmus while passing stool but excreta is extremely hard and passed in minimal quantity: Colo cynth.
- Weeps continuosly day and night: Psorinum.
- Sleep well upto sunrise but continues to weep till noon time: Calcarea Carb.

- Weeps due to locking up of wind in the stomach (in relation to cyanosis of whole body): Calc.Carb.
- Bores his head into the pillow and places his hand behind his ear: Bryonia.
- Suddenly weeps and also suddenly stops weeping: Belladonna.
- Weeps while being forcibly fed by mother: Calc Phos.
- Weeps due to some apparent and visible cause: Causticum.
- Weeps due to worms distended abdomen alongwith pain in the stomach: Staphysagria.
- Weeps due to ill- effects of anger: Aconite.
- Weeps due to retarded growth of limbs: Lyco, Magn. Mur
- Weeps due to fear of going down: Borax.
- Weeps due to fear of movement. Wishes to be carried in Rhus Tox, Cina
- Child cries in pauses (not continuously): Apis.
- Child cries in a heart-rending voice: Cuprum Met.
- Child cries during the time of sleep: Cina.
- Child cries during/at the time of teething: Aethusa, Natum Mur, Mag. Phos.
- Child cries and continues to cry even when looked up casually and gets up agitated after sleep: Antim.Tart.
- Child passes blood from Nose: Terebinthina.

- Does not wish to feed with milk. Cod liver Oil.
- Child sees odd thing and weeps: Aethusa.
- Child weeps unless holded: Chamom.

Note: Initially, if you find any symptom, give single medicine in 30 potency, one or two drops, thrice a day in one spoon of water. If there is no response, consult a qualified, experienced homeoathic physician.

10

BIOCHEMIC COMBINATION TABLETS

Biochemic remedies were invented by great scientist Schussler of Germany. Here are the details of 28 Bio-Combinations:

Bio-Plasgen No.1

Anaemia

Composition:

Calc. Phos, Ferr. Phos, Nat Mur and Kali phos.

Diseases Covered:

Lack of blood due to indigestible food and due to living in unhealthy quarters. Cerebral and spinal anaemia, continuous loss of blood from any part of body. A general wasting of the tissues. Waxy appearance of skin, chlorosis. Palpitation, tremor and weakness. Anaemia of the brain due to prolonged mental strain.

Dosage:

Adults 4 tablets, children 2 tablets at a time, at an interval of 3-4 hours daily.

Bio-Plasgen No.2

Asthma.

Components:

Kali ars, Magn. ars, Nat Mur and Nat Sulph.

Symptoms:

Nervous asthma accompanied by cough, gasping, irregular pulse. Asthma with troublesome flatulence or spasms. Tickling and convulsive cough. Bronchial asthma with yellow sputum. Better in cool/open air, worse towards evening and in warm rooms.

Dosage:

Adults 4 tablets, children 2 tablets, at a time, 4 times daily.

Bio-Plasgen No.3

Colic

Components:

Calc Phos, Ferr. Phos, Magn. Phos and Calc. Sulph.

Symptoms:

Colic of children and adults from blockade of the intestines caused by flatulence or constipation with formation of gas. Colics of infants, compelling them to draw up their legs. Spasmodic pains of adults too, causing the patient to double up.

Bio-Plasgen No.4

Constipation

Components

Calc. Flour, Kali Mur, Natr. Mur and Silicea.

Symptoms

Constipated bowels without any apparent cause. Stools dry, hard and black. Liver torpid. Dull headache, foul breath, tongue coated; bad taste in mouth.

Dosage

Adults 4 tablets. Children 2 tablets, at a time, 4 times daily.

Bio-Plasgen No.5

Coryza

Components

Ferr. Phos, Kali Sulph and Natr Mur.

Symptoms

Sneezing, continuous thick white discharge from the nose or discharge from bronchial tubes due to an irritation and severe inflammation of the mucus membranes. Pain in the head and fever. Tongue is grey/white coated.

Dosage

Adults 4 tablets and children 2 tablets daily at an interval of 4 hours (4 doses daily).

Bio-Plasgen No.6

Cough, Cold and Catarrh

Components

Ferr Phos, Kali Mur, Magn. Phos, Nat Mur, Nat Sulph.

Symptoms

Cold in the head, acute catarrh, hollow cough that rattles, respiration with pain in chest, bronchitis.

Dosage

Adults 4 tablets and children 2 tablets daily at an internal of 4 hours. (4 doses daily)

Bio-Plasgen No.7

Diabetes [Suitable for insipidus and mellitus conditions.]

Components

Calc Phos, Ferr. Phos, Kali Sulph, Nat. Phos and Nat. Sulph.

Symptoms

Increased malnutrition, pain in calves, excessive thirst, dryness of lips. Nervous prostration and sleeplessness. Suits all chronic cases where the liver is disordered. A useful remedy to support the patient's general health by assimilating the glucose. Also improves impaired Kidney and nerve functions adversely affected by diabetes.

Dosage

Adults 4 tablets and children 2 tablets. 4 times daily.

Bio-Plasgen No.8

Diarrhoea

Components

Calc. Phos, Ferr. Phos, Kali Phos, Kali Sulph, Nat. Sulph.

Symptoms

Thin watery stools with undigested food, thirst caused by fat or too rich food. Tongue white-coated. Prostration. More beneficial in convalescence period.

Dosage

Adults 4 tablets and children 2 tablets. 4 times daily.

Bio-Plasgen No.9

Dysentry

Components

Ferr. Phos, Kali Mur., Kali Phos, Magn. Phos.

Symptoms

Pain when stools begin to pass which contain blood and mucus. Patient feels a constant urge to empty his stomach.

Dosage

Adults 4 tablets and children 2 tablets. 4 times daily.

Bio-Plasgen No. 10

Enlarged Tonsils

Components

Calc. Phos, Fer. Phos, Kali Mur.

Symptoms

Fever and a feeling of lassitude. Pain in the back and limbs. Throat lined with a white lining. Tonsils swollen. Bad breath, tongue coated, no appetite.

Dosage

Adults 4 tablets and children 2 tablets. 4 times daily.

Bio-Plasgen No. 11

Fever

Components:

Ferr. Phos, Kali Mur, Kali Sulph, Nat. Mur, Nat Sulph.

Symptoms

Useful in all kinds of fever and chill, initial stages of inflammatory diseases. In quick sudden swellings. pneumonic, pleurisy and other inflammatory conditions that tend to or cause suppuration.

Dosage

Adults 4 tablets and children 2 tablets. 4 times daily.

Bio-Plasgen No. 12

Headache

Components

Ferr. phos, Kali phos, Magn. Phos, Nat Mur.

Symptoms

Headaches due to congestion and rush of blood to head. Neuralgia. Worse from cold but better (relief) from heat. Nervousness as a consequence of worries. Sleeplessness and/or low-functioning of the liver. Headache is better in the open air but worse in the evening or in a warm room.

Dosage

Adults 4 tablets and children 2 tablets. 4 times daily.

Bio-Plasgen No. 13

Leucorrhoea [Popularly known as 'The whites'].

Components

Calc. phos, Nat Mur, Kali phos, Kali Sulph.

Symptoms

Useful in all forms and stages, that is during puberty, pregnancy and in the climacteric, in states of general weakness and hysteria.

Dosage

Adults 4 tablets 4 times daily.

Bio-Plasgen No. 14

Measles

Components

Ferr phos, Kali M7ur, Kali phos.

Symptoms

Sneezing, discharge from nose, watery eyes and fever. It is useful in all stages.

Dosage

Adults 4 tablets and children 2 tablets 4 times daily.

Bio-Plasgen No. 15

Menstruation Troubles.

Components

Calc. phos, Ferr. phos, Kali phos, Kali Sulph, Magn phos.

Symptoms

Menses are irregular and painful; scanty and late in young women. Menses too early, last longer and flow is profuse, particularly in middle-aged women.

Dosage

Adults 4 tablets and children 2 tablets. 4 times daily.

Bio-Plasgen No. 16

Nervous Exhaustion

Components

Calc phos, Ferr phos, Kali phos, Magn phos, Nat. phos.

Symptoms

Fatigue and nervous exhaustion from whichever cause. A general weakness of the heart, stomach and nervous system. Nervousness.

Dosage

Adults 4 tablets and children 2 tablets 4 times daily.

Bio-Plasgen No. 17

Colic

Components

Calc. Fluor, Ferr Phos, Kali Phos, Kali Mur.

Symptoms

It is a useful remedy against all haemorrhoidal knots and cures all kinds of piles. External piles with stinging pains; bleeding piles without or with pain.

Dosage

Adults 4 tablets and children 2 tablets, 4 times daily.

Bio-Plasgen No. 18

Pyorrhoea

Components

Calc. Fluor, Calc. Sulph, Silicea.

Symptoms

Gums bleed easily, are spongy, inflammed and swollen. Pus in the gums, Breath foul.

Dosage

Adults 4 tablets and children 2 tablets, 4 times daily.

Bio-Plasgen No. 19

Rheumatism

Components

Ferr. Phos, Kali Sulph, Magn. Phos, Nat. Sulph.

Symptoms

Useful in lumbago, sciatica, muscular rheumatism, shooting and stabbing pains in the points of arms and legs.

Dosage

Adults 4 tablets and children 2 tablets, 4 times daily.

Bio-Plasgen No. 20

Skin Diseases

Components

Calc. Fluor, Calc. Sulph, Kali Sulph, Nat. Mur, Nat. Sulph.

Symptoms

Acne, herpes, pemphigus, crusta lactea and similar eruptive diseases. Eczema due to disorders of the uterus. Scurfy eruptions on the scalp and in the faces of children.

Dosage

Adults 4 tablets and children 2 tablets, 4 times daily.

Bio-Plasgen No. 21

Teething Troubles of Babies

Components

Calc. Phos, Ferr. Phos.

Symptoms

Children cry, are naughty and obstinate during time of teething. The formulation helps the children in cutting teeth easily and quickly by supplying important salts to the babies. Their digestion is improved and appetite is also improved. Tablets build up babies and improve their general health and abolish griping.

Dosage

2 tablets 4 times daily.

Bio-Plasgen No. 22

Scrofula

Components

Calc. Phos, Ferrum Phos, Kali Mur, Silicea.

Symptoms

Relieves both dry and suppurating glandular abscesses. The compound covers almost all the symptoms of the disease.

Dosage

Adults 4 tablets and children 2 tablets, 4 times daily.

Bio-Plasgen No. 23

Toothache

Components

Calc. Fluor, Ferr. Phos, Magn. Phos.

Symptoms

Useful especially in neuralgic cases. Also has favourable effect in rheumatic toothache.

Dosage

4 tablets for adults, 2 tablets for children to be given 4 times daily or as and when required.

Bio-Plasgen No. 24

Tonic for the nerves and brain

Components

Calc. Phos, Ferr. Phos, Kali Phos, Mag. Phos; Nat. Phos.

Symptoms

Suitable as a general tonic for all chronically wasting diseases; anaemia of quickly growing young people. Very useful for women who have been rendered weak by frequent child-bearing, general debility and exhaustion with a lack of vitality.

Dosage

4 tablets for adults and 2 tablets for children, 4 times daily.

Bio-Plasgen No. 25

Acidity, Flatulence and Indigestion

Components

Nat. Phos, Nat. Sulph, Silicea.

Symptoms

Gastric disturbances, flatulence, acidity, dyspepsia, acid and sour risings; feeling or weight in abdomen, bilious vomiting; colics, flatulence and headache.

Dosage

4 tablets for adults and 2 tablets for children, 4 times daily.

Bio-Plasgen No. 26

Easy delivery/parturition

Components

Calc. Phos, Calc. Fluor, Kali Phos; Magn. Phos.

Symptoms

These tablets, if taken during the entire period of pregnancy, will greatly relieve pains of labour. They also ensure general health and well-being of the expectant mother, in addition to assisting in the health and development of the child (infant). They might also prevent miscarriage.

Dosage

4 tablets 4 times daily.

Bio-Plasgen No. 27

Lack of Vitality

Components

Calc. phos, Kali phos, Nat. Mur.

Symptoms

Impotence; depression of sexual instinct, general debility and lassitude, emissions followed by weakness and trembling. Too early aging. It virtually tones up entire sexual system.

Dosage

4 tablets, 4 times daily.

Bio-Plasgen No. 28

General Tonic

Components

All the twelve tissue Remedies. This is combination of all the twelve tissue remedies found in the human organism. The tablets are of great help for those persons who suffer from consumption and other debilitating and wasting diseases; for convalescence from fever, diarrhoea, pneumonia, etc. because they help to build up the system by supplying requisite and necessary tissue nutrition. Old and weak persons should take them daily after meals to derive tonic effects. Its continuous use will ward off chances of disease by building up general resistance of the body.

Dosage

2 Tablets 3 to 4 times daily - half an hour before or after meals and also at bed-time.

Note: Quantities and concentrations of various tissue salts used in above mentioned preparations are based on research, testing and experiences of the formulators and practitioners, as such they should be taken, as sold in the market (but reliability must be ensured) and should be purchased as sealed vials only of reputed homoeopathic manufactures like WSI, SBL, Bakson, Ralson, Bioforce, Beck & Koll, Reckeveg etc.

11

CONSTIPATION AND ITS TREATMENT

Constipation is a condition in which the bowels are evacuated at a longer interval or with difficulty. What the right interval should be, is difficult to generalize since it varies from person to person. Some evacuate their bowels once, others twice a day, while there are others who seek this pleasure only once in 2 or 3 days and yet have sound health.

What Causes Constipation?

Some may have constipation on account of the change of enviornment, or emotional tension, but the normal rhythm returns after a few days, and should not be a source of worry. The most important causes of constipation are a disregard of the call to pass motion and an improper diet. When the rectum is full, it sends signals to the intestines through the central nervous system for their movement and if this is repeatedly ignored it gradually leads to failure of the rectum to signal the urge. The diet should contain a reasonable amount of non absorbable material to form a bulk which acts as a stimulus for the intestinal movements. Highly spicy foodstuffs such as chaat, pickles and hot curries may stimulate the bowel to cause a complete evacuation, but this is followed by inactivity of the intestines and constipation. Slimilarly, purgatives also stimulate the intestines, to cause their evacuation and this is also followed by constipation. To treat this constipation, again a purgative is needed and this continues in the form of a constipation purgative constipation cycle. Other causes of constipation may be a disease or abnormality of gastrointestinal tract, adverse effects of drugs, drying of the stools (faecal impaction), obstruction of the intestines, and severe illness in which food intake is too small. In case of prolonged constipation in the infants or intermittent constipation with diarrhoea, the physician should be consulted to rule out surgical problems.

What Can Be Done About Constipation?

If you are suffering from constipation, and have been taking purgative, try to stop these gradually. Your system will probably return to normal if you take enough soups, vegetables, fruits etc. However, if you are the worrying type you may take milk laxative only as a temporary measure without making it a habit. Remember, disregarding the call for motion is the worst you can do to your consipation. Do not wait unnecessarily. Rush to the toilet wherever you are, whether at a party or in the kitchen. Your diets should be made up of high roughage foods containing a lot of whole grain cereals, leafy vegetables like spinach, raw carrots and cucumbers, salads, prunes, figs, papaya, water melon and other fresh fruits. Your intestines will soon gain the normal tone. If all these measures fail, you are a candidate for milk purgatives or laxatives. Never take strong purgatives. They are needed only under exceptional circumstances and should be used under the care of a doctor. The purgatives which are commonly used are described here.

Mild Purgatives

Mild purgatives or laxatives are those which promote defecation causing minimum adverse effects. Drugs included in this group are:

Bulk Producing Drugs

Isapgol (sat Isabgol), Agar-agar (Agarol), Methyle celluslose.

These drugs absorb water to increase the bulk in the intestines and make the stools soft. The onset of their action is slow, about 12 to 24 hours. They are the safest purgatives for the treatment of chronic constipation. Of the three, isapgol is most commonly used in our country.

Dosage

Isapgol is given preferably with warm milk in a dose of 4 to 5 g once or twice a day. Agar-agar is given in a dose of 4 to 16 g and methyl cellulose in 1 to 6 g in divided doses, for children in the age group of 12-15 years. For younger children the dose should be half.

Adverse Effects

Those agents which are derived from vegetable sources are devoid of toxic effects. Occasionally flatulence may occur, but, this can be relieved by increasing the fluid intake. The chronic use of isapgol may decrease plasma cholesterol by interfering with the absorption of bile acids but it does not cause any harm and may rather do good to an obese patient.

Precaution

Always take plenty of fluids along with these drugs to obtain maximum benefit and to avoid the possibility of intestinal obstruction which has been reported to occur in rare cases.

Stool Softeners

Dioctyle Sodium Sulfosuccinate

This is an effective stool softener for the treatment of constipation in some cases. It is a detergent which absorbs water by reducing the surface tension of fluids in the stools.

Dosage

The daily dose varies from 50 to 500mg depending on the severity of the condition. The action starts after 24 to 48 hours.

Adverse Effects

Adverse effects of this drug are quite rare. It has been reported to interact with mineral oils to increase their absorption.

Precaution

It should not be taken with mineral oils.

Liquid Paraffin (Cremaffin)

This is a traditional remedy for constipation. It is an inert oil which lubricates the intestines and forms a film or coating around the stools to make its passage smooth and comfortable. It softens the stool by preventing the absorption of water into the intestines. It is often recommended to patients of piles, heart attack, and to pregnant women, as well as after surgery on the rectum or abdomen and in cases in which straining to evacuate may be harmful. It is quite popular as it allows the stool to pass through the intestines with a minimum of friction.

Dosage

Liquid paraffin is given in a dose of 15 to 45 ml. Its action starts after 12 to 24 hours.

Adverse Effects

If taken regularly, it may cause deficiency of fat soluble Vitamins such as A, D and K. It may at times leak through the gastrointestinal tract and cause not only annoying but embarrassing situation. Its presence in the rectum inhibits the stimulatory reflexes to the intestines and prevents complete evacuation of bowels. On aspiration, liquid paraffin has also been reported to cause lipoid pneumonia in elderly and weak persons. Although it promotes and facilitates the passage of stools, it delays healing and, therefore, its use is not preferred after surgery for piles.

Precautions

1. It should not be taken regularly as it may cause deficiency of Vitamins A, D and K . This may be very harmful, specially in pregnant women.
2. It should not be taken by very old and weak persons, and young children because of the danger of lipoid pneumonia.
3. It should not be taken during the day time because of chances of its leakage through the rectum.
4. It delays healing, and is not recommended after an operation on piles.
5. It should not be taken along with dioctyls sodium sulfosuccinate, as the latter promotes its absorption from the intestines.

Mild Saline Purgatives

Magnesium Hydroxide

This is a mild laxative which can be used even by pregnant women and children. It absorbs water from the intestines to form the bulk and make the stools soft. Besides purgative action, it counteracts acidity in the stomach.

Dosage

Its usual dose is 2 to 4g. its action starts after 2 to 6 hours.

Adverse Effects

It is a mild purgative and does not have any adverse effect except to produce flatulence in some people.

Precautions

1. Take plenty of fluids along with this purgative.
2. Patients with chronic kidney disease who may have difficulty in excreting magnesium should be wary of milk of Magnesia.

Sodium Potassium Tartrate

It is the basic ingredient of commonly used ENO's fruit salt and Seidlitz powder. These also contain tartaric acid and sodium bicarbonate which interact to produce carbondioxide gas, forming an effervescent drink, which resembles gas containing soft drinks. The gas present in the solution distends the stomach and reflexly stimulates movements of the intestines. It also absorbs water from the intestines which assists in forming the bulk and softening the stools.

Dosage

The dose of sodium potassium tartrate for its purgative action is 10g. Its action starts after 3 to 6 hours.

Adverse Effects

Sodium potassium tartrate is a safe purgative and does not cause any adverse effect.

Precautions

It should not be taken by those who are on a sodium restricted diet, e.g. patients of heart failure, hypertension etc, but children are free of all such problems.

Note: The dose should be half of the prescribed dose and keep in touch with your paediatrician.

12

HOMOEOPATHIC TREATMENT OF ASTHMA

Homoeopathy is based on symptom similatrity.

Senega-Q

Give 5-6 drops in water when Ipecac, Ars or Lobelia have failed to yield results. It is best when cough, at first, is dry later on cough with excessive expectoration, wheezing sound pain and sense of constriction in the chest, rattling noise with chest; loss of voice, on ascending during rest and while moving in the open air. When sweat appears and when head is lowered. Voice unsteady, partial paralysis of vocal cords, sore chest walls, even profuse mucus difficult to raise up, feeling as if lungs were forced back to spine. Also useful when cough ends up in a sneeze.

Blata Orient-Q

Give 5-6 drops in water, either just before appearace of symptoms, on the outset or even during attack. It will shorten asthmatic attack's duration and give relief. Asthma with bronchitis. Cough with laboured breathing. Mucus resembles like pus. Suited best to robust, stout and obese (fat) persons. Stop its use when improvement is seen, otherwise it will cause recurrence of symptoms.

Lobelia Inflat-Q

Any exertion, by rapid walking, feeling as if heart would stop beating, sensation of weight and pressure on the chest, Asthmatic attacks with much weakness–especially felt in pit of stomach and preceeded by prickling all over. Cramps, dyspnoea from constriction of chest, ringing cough and short breath, catches his throat to seek relief, emphysema of the aged person, after use of tobacco towards evening and from warmth. Dose same as for above-mentioned medicines.

Eridictyon-Q or 3x

Asthma relieved by expectoration, bronchial pthisis, with night sweats and emaciation, cough after influenza, wheezing sounds, coryza, dull pain in right lung. Appetite poor and defective digestion. Whooping cough symptoms.

Give 5-20 drops in water, according to severity of symptoms. Avoid repeating quiete often.

Eucalyptus-G-Q

Enlarged and ulcerated and inflamed throat and tonsils. Asthma with dyspnoea and palpitation. Moist Asthma, expectoration white and mucus thick. Bronchial affections of old people. Profuse muco-pus expertoration which is of offensive character. Irritative cough. Whooping cough (expecially of rachitic children). Foetid form of bronchitis, bronchial dialation and emphysema.

Spread 4-5 drops on a piece of cotton or some cloth (say handkerchief) and let the patient inhale. Some mother tincture may also be orally taken, as and when felt necessary (8-10 drops in water).

When an attack of asthma has abated, it is better to place the patient under treatment and close supervision of qualified physician whose services and advise should be freely and easily available in both acute (emergent) stages and for inter-paroxysimnal treatment.

13

CURE OF HYPERTENTION

(Holistic Therapies and Homoeopathy)

To properly understand what hypertention is, it is essential to know something about blood, blood vesels and the circulatory system.

Hypertention is the disorder of the blood vessels. The blood circulating in the body through the blood vessels (arteries) supplies oxygen as well as nourshiment to all existing cells in the system. The heart pumps blood into the large arteries. The pumping created by this pressure is the blood presure. For the circulation of blood, pressure-up to a certain limit is essential. When this normal pressure increases a little, the smaller blood vessels narrow down forcing the heart to pump blood with grater effort. Hence the blood pressure rises in proportion to the heart's pressure. The heart has to beat faster and exert pressure to supply blood to various organs resulting in the pressure getting high and giving rise to hypertention.

How and Why is it caused?

Though many factors may bring about hypertention, overeating with the resultant obsesity is a very common cause. Another important and familiar cause is stress of all types. Hypertention caused by stress is aggravated and defiles complete cure, when intake of tobacco and alcohal also exists. A single cigratte raises the systolic pressure five to ten points, temporarily. But in cases of chain smoking, it will keep the pressure raised.

Some infectious diseases, such as tonsils and typhoid in childhood, sometimes impare the functioning of the kidney in later years, causing high blood pressure, in such cases it should be considered as a natural compensatory mechanism to maintain a normal filtration rate through the hardened walls of the small blood vessels in the kidney, which otherwise results in worsening of kidney disorders.

Many young women suffer from hypertention due to the attack of convulsions during pregnancy, known as eclampsia and other kidney disorders of pregenacy associate with an elevated blood pressure. Mental stress, when prolonged without respite, may rise the blood pressure permanentaly without its coming down even after the stress is removed.

Excessive intake of coffee, tea, cola drinks, refined food, pain killer, excessive salt, a high-fat low-fiber diet and processed food, which does not contain essential nutrients, prevent the explusion of waase and toxic matter from the body, due to which the blood vessels become slack.

Hydrothreapy

Hot foot bath: this is the most useful and effective of water treatment for many diseases. It is used with other forms of the treatment to make them more effective. Whenever, foot-bath is given, it is necessary to give a cold compress on the head. this will bring relief quickly and prevent any possibility of giddiness.

Method

Fill a tub with hot water upto ankles. The tempreature of the water should suit the individual's tolerance. The duration of bath should be from 10 to 20 minutes. At the end of the bath, the feet must be rubbed with a towel wet in cold water or should be splashed with cold water. Afterwards the feet should be dried briskly with a thick towel.

Hot foot bath dilates the blood vessels of the skin in the feet and draws the blood run from the congeated part of the body. It cures many diseases such as headaches of all origin, insomnia, fatigue, mental tiredness, coldness of the extremities, poor blood circulation and rheumatism etc.

Diet Plan

Break fast (7 to 9 A.M.)

1. Orange juice or any fruit juice or sweet orange or mausambi: One Cup
2. Fresh apple or any fresh fruit (except mangoes and lichi): One
3. Germinated gram 1/4 cup
4. Wheat bread with green vegetable ot toast: As desired
5. Skimmed milk (if desired): One cup

Lunch and Dinner (12 to 2 P.M. 6 to 8 P.M.)

1. Salad: Mixture of tomato, cucumber, radish, lettuce, carrot etc. with very little salt and lemon juice or with french dressing or plain: One cup
2. Vegetable Soup: One cup
3. Wheat bread: As desired
4. Pulse: As desired
5. Saag: As desired
6. Green vegetable of any kind fish for Non-Vegetarians: 2 pieces.

After noon Refreshment (3 to 5 p.m.)

1. Fresh fruit of any type: As desired
2. Salted biscuits or chana ghughani: As desired

The important points to be kept in mind are the major part of every day diet should be of Salad, Fresh fruit and green vegetables. Dishes should be cooked in vegetable oils by using no spices or very little of it.

Garlic and onion are useful foods for blood pressure due to presence of ' Fibroletic' element which helps in clothing process and mulsification of blood which are natural traits of blood chemistry, apart from restoring blood to normal (by processing of liquification.) Do not use salt in blood pressure; as lesser/ trapered consumption of salt will provide much relief.

Breathing exercises 1

Sit in a comfortable position with crossed legs. Keep the body relaxed and erect. Keep the mouth closed. Inhale fast as much air as possible and exhale quickly with force. Do not hold the breathe but breathe in and out in quick sugession. Relax a while, breathing normally and again start breathing in and out quick in succession. Do this five to six times in the beginning and slowly increase after a few day's practice.

Breathing exercise 2

Sit cross-legged on the ground or on a chair or stand with folded hands as in prayer. Keep mouth closed and breathe in through the nostril counting one to four. Hold breath till you count from five to eight. Start to breathe out. While breathing out count once again one to four, hold breath till you count five to eight before you start inhaling. Repeat this a few more times. Increase the number of counts while breathing in and out and in between, gradually from day to day, to draw in more oxygen and expel more carbon-dioxide.

Breathing Exercise 3

Sit cross-legged on the ground or on a chair with the spine erect and muscles relaxed . Cover the right nostril with the thumb and inhale through the left nostril. Cover the left nostril too with the index finger and hold down the breath for 1 or 2 counts. Release the thumb and exhale through the right nostril. Repeat this with the left nostril. Cover the left nostril with the index finger and inhale through the right. Close both the nostril and hold for 1 or 2 counts and then exhale through the left nostril releasing the index finger. With regular practice the number of counts while holding the breath should increase.

This exercise corrects the disorders of the nasal cavity and lungs. The good supply of oxygen helps purify the lungs.

Those who suffer from blood pressure must not practice to hold the breath. They can simply inhale and exhale.

Shitali Pranayama

1. Sit in Padmasana.
2. Open your lips like a break of crow and protrude your tongue and fold it in the middle.
3. Inhale through the tongue slowly and fill air in belly.
4. Retain for a few seconds and exhale through both nostril.
5. Repeat five to ten times.

Precuation

This Pranayama produces coldness, therefore it is not to be practiced in very cold weather or people suffering from colds.

Benefits

It reduces high blood pressure and purifies the blood.

Sheetkari Pranayama

1. Sit in padmasana.
2. Bring your tongue near your teeth so as to touch them.
3. With a little gap between the teeth inhale slowly and fill belly with air.
4. Exhale through both the nostrils.

Benefits

Reduce blood presserve and purifies the blood.

Shava Asana

Lie down on your back. Keep whole body loose and in a straight position. Palms can be either on the floor or you can keep them upwardly. Do not use any pillow under your head. At this point keep breathing in normal way. Keep the eyes closed and let the whole body fall on the floor in an unrestrained way. This is the position during the actual practice.

Steps for practice

1. Close your eyes and keep them closed for two seconds. Then open them for two seconds. Do this simple opening and closing of eyes for three to four times.
2. Open the eyes again and look upward, then downward then straight. Now look towards the left side, then towards the right side, then straight again and then close the eyes. Repeat this eyes exercise two to three times.
3. Now open your mouth wide without straining it. Turn the tongue inside the mouth in such a way that its tip is

folded backward in the throat area, then close the mouth. Keep the mouth closed and tongue folded for 10 seconds. Then open the mouth and bring the tongue back to its normal position, then close the mouth. Repat the process for 2 to 3 times.

4. Keeping your eyes closed, bring your mental attention towards your toes. See (mentally) that the toes are relaxed. Then move slowly upwards and towards the head area mentally by checking the knees, thighs, waist, spinal cord, back, shoulders, neck, arms, palms, fingers and rest of the area of the body to be sure that they are actually relaxed. Make a slight movement of the neck and head by turning right and left. Then let the head rest at a comfortable position. Now the entire body is physically relaxed.
5. Then relax the mind with the following process: Select a place of natural beauty which you have ever visited and liked, such as park, a garden, a lawn or a riverside and feel as if you are mentally present at that place. Attach your mind to that place . Feel as if you are lying at that place and breathing air of the same environment. Now while keeping the mind involved with that environment, do some deep breathing . In this deep breathing, just exhale and inhale slowly but deeply. During the breathing, the stomach should go upward while inhaling and it should come downward while exhaling. One exhalatation and one inhalation make one round. Do not rush in this deep breathing. Make about ten to twelve rounds. When the deep breathing is over, feel as if you are going to sleep. Now relax completly. Stay in that position for 5 to 10 minutes. Then open your eyes and stretch your body and then be seated. You have completed the Shavasana.

Benefits

Shavasana has a very good effect upon the patient as well as upon any yoga practioner. One immediate effect is that it relaxes all the muscles, nerves and the organ of the body system. When the muscles, nerves and the organs are fully relaxed, they gain strength and their normal health is restored.

For the people suffering from insomnia, high and low blood pressure, gastric trouble, lungs and heart troubles and mental sickness, Shavasana is a remarkable kriya for providing immediate relief. Beside all these exercise padmasana, bhujangasana, parvatasana and suptvajrasana are benefited in hypertension.

Acupressure Treatment

Make pressure on left foot and left hand by your thumb on palm and sole in between first finger and thumb. These are the trigger points to keep the heart fit. Apart from these points there are certain points on left and right hand on outer surface of little fingers below the root of nail. Daily for one minute in fractions of 15-20 seconds, pressure should be given on these points to combat hypertension.

Magneto Therapy

- Wear magnetic wrist band on right wrist to avoid high B.P.
- Keep a ceramic or low power magnet on your forehead.
- Keep north pole of a low power magnet behind right to control hypertension.
- Drink magnetic water, a cup, twice a day.

Colour Therapy

Out of the reasons that trigger hypertension is rise in cholestrol level and if this is the sole cause of the disease in that case ingest a cup of green water twice daily–once after each meal. If cause be renal malfunctioning, then green water should be taken thrice daily, because use of green water restores normal functioning of kidneys. It is a magical medicine for kidney.

Gem Theraphy

Ruby, corundum, coral and high quality pearls are the best stone. If a high quality ruby of Burmese origin is worn in healthy condition, no rise in blood pressur will ever occur, as it is a godly gift for the disease because it controls blood circulation.

Homoeopathic Therapy

Homoeopathy is based on symptom similarity. On the basis of totality of symptoms these medicines can be used after consultation from an experienced Homoeopathic Physicians -

- Passiflora Q
- Rauvolfia Q
- Belladona 30
- Cactus G 30
- Creatagus Q
- Nux Vomica 200

There are certain other remedies which can be used as per symptoms of the patient.

14

ATTRACTION OF FACE

The whole body is kept covered with clothes, but face is a part left open and exposed to summer, winter and rains. So you must care for it.The face is the mirror of your mind and whole body.

Beauty was a mere blessing in olden times. Being beautiful or ugly was taken matter of fate. But today it has become an art with aid of cosmetics. Any lady can be perfect in this by making sincere efforts.

Not that everyone has sharp features and fair complexion. Make up can hide many of the deficiencies. If you have a strong will, no one can stop you from becoming beautiful.

A lady good in make-up can hide her deficiencies and be beautiful, whereas another one may be normal but can look unpleasant without proper make-up.

But make-up will glow a face which is healthy. Can all this blossom on a sick, glowless, plae, dull face? Never. So, first improve your health to have a beautiful face.

Besides Smoothie, take balanced and nutritious food for good health so that you possess it forever.

Exercise:

A few exercises are being explained below for the face. They are very easy. They will exercise muscles of the face and it will glow.

It will not hang loose, or get disproportionate but shall remain rather musclar.

- Pull both corners of lips with fingers. Count one to ten. The upper lip should touch the lower one must not turn outwards. It makes lower portion of the face shapeful. It brings a balance in the shape of the face.
- Fill your mouth with air and move it up-down in round motion for three minutes. It will improve blood circulation and dullness will vanish.
- Keep pressing the corners of the lips. Keep the face like this for three minutes. Movement of cheeks as well as jaw will improve the shape.
- Massage your cheeks with the hands from down upwards and outwards and repeat it ten times. It will improve the shape and bring glow on the cheeks.

ACNE & PIMPLES

There are a common inflammatory disorders of the sebaceous glands just below the skin surface and characterized by the recurring formation of black heads, white heads and pimples.

Acne

Primarily, acne occurs on the face but in some cases, it may be noticed on the back, shoulders, chest and arms.

Causes

Hormones

The culprits are at their peak of activity thus influencing the secretion of the sebaceous glands. The excess production of sebum causes breakouts that are highly incident during puberty and menstruation. At times, psychological stress causes acne.

Cleanse skin morning and night with milk or home-made cleansers. Refrain from using facial scrub, when acne is severe. Stop picking your pimples and acne.

Diet is an important factor in acne.

Balanced nutrition and diet, skin hygiene, adequate sleep, exercise, fresh air and sunlight help in combating acne.

Carbohydrates and foods with a high fat content should be avoided from diet.

Increase fiber intake and water to avoid constipation, which is also a causative factor for acne.

The high content of oxalic acid that is present in chocolates, coca and rhubarb inhibit the body's absorption of calcium. Since calcium maintains the acid-alkali balance of the body, it is important for a clear complexion.

Reducing salt intake in your diet also shows a remarkable improvement in complexion. Vitamins are necessary for your lovely, smooth skin.

Vitamin A is important for clear, healthy skin.

Vitamin B complex reduces facial greasiness and the formation of blackheads.

Combating Acne

- Saturate cotton wool in mint juice extract and apply every day.
- Apply crushed marigold leaves on acne.
- Boil and mash plums to get roughly eight teaspoons. Combine with one teaspoon of almond oil and apply.
- Make a smooth paste of Kasturi Turmeric and apply evenly on acne.

- Apply a mask made out of fresh Azadiracta (neem) leaves ground to a fine paste. Add ¼ teaspoon of turmeric powder, sandal wood paste and gram flour. Let it dry completely before rinsing.

Banishing Pimples

- Swab face with camphor lotion on pimples daily. Wash off with medicated soap and lukewarm water.
- Grind mint leaves to extract pure juice. Apply generously and allow it to dry, before washing off.
- Sandal wood ground to a paste using undiluted cucumber juice may be used.
- One tablespoon of gram flour, half teaspoon of turmeric powder, one teaspoon of neem juice and enough milk to make a smooth consistency. Leave on for twenty minutes before washing off.
- Pimples can vanish overnight if you rub a little starch paste on the pimple at bedtime.

SUNBURN & FRECKLES

It has been rightly remarked that "sun can be woman's best friend or her worst enemy". Sun in moderation, lights up your beauty and excess exposure to sun gives your skin the look of old leather.

Sun Burn

Sunlight is excellent for you as it is nature's source of vitamin D. Strong sunlight over prolonged periods are best avoided as it leads to sunburn. Your skin produces melanin which acts as an in-built barrier against ultra violet rays.

Over exposure to sun, causes to UV rays to actually burn up surface skin and penetrate deep into lower cells causing sunburn and other aging problems like lines and wrinkles.

Sunburn is a condition that is better prevented than treated. Sunburn can be a painful affair literally.

Despite your intentions, if you are a victim of sunburn, pamper your skin with

(a) Application of vitamin D ointment.

(b) Use peanut oil, olive oil or lanolin.

(c) Mineral oil can also be used.

AIDS FROM KITCHEN

- Drink plenty of lemon juice before venturing outdoors.
- Grate and squeeze cucumber. Spread the seeds and juice over the burn.
- Take three small tomatoes and mash well. Add a cup of butter milk. Mix well and apply on skin. Allow to dry for one hour atleast.

  This will help to reduce pain and take heat out of skin.
- Cold water compresses together with an additional intake of vitamin A, C and E are recommended for the treatment of sunburn.

(d) Anti-sunburn lotion

Ingredients

1 lemon

1 egg white

Method

Add juice of lemon to the white of egg. Mix briskly, transfer contents to a pan and simmer on low fire till it thickens. Cool it.

Apply to sunburn and do not wash off.

- Boil lettuce leaves in a cup of boiling water to get a strong infusion which may be applied on sunburn skin.
- Use whey on your sunburn.
- Yoghurt together with little honey helps to cool and promote healing in sunburnt skin.
- Combine together a teaspoon of lemon juice with 7-8 drops of milk and gently massage on to skin. Let it soak in before rinsing off with soap and water.

15

REMEDIES FOR BRUISES, SPRAINS, STRAINS, WOUNDS

REMEDIES FOR BRUISES

Remedies	Specific Indications	Worse From	Better From
Arnica (Internally or lotion)	Common bruises, injuries from blow or fall, Shock	Least touch, Rest	Lying down, Head low
Hypericum (Internally or lotion)	Crushing injuries to nerves, Nerve injury to:"Crazybones", Fingertips, Nailbeds, Palms, Soles of feet, Tailbones, Toes, Puncture wounds	Cold, Touch	
Ledum (Internally or lotion)	Bruises: Cold and numb bruised parts, Long-lasting Black eye, Splinter under nail, Bruised nerves, Puncture wounds	Warmth	Bathing in cold water
Ruta	Injuries of: Bones, Periosteum, bone covering, Shins, Soft tissue, Prolapsed, protruding rectum, Wrist and ankle sprains	Lying down, Cold,wet weather	

SPRAINS

Remedies	General Indications	First-Aid Measures
Arnica (Internally or lotion)	Shock of injury, Bleeding in tissues	Massage injured area gently with *Arnica* oil or lotion, but only on unbroken skin. Elevate injured part. During the first 24 hours, apply ice bag or cold compress to painful area to reduce swelling and pain; apply heat after that. Wrap injured area with elastic bandage for support.
Bryonia	Injured joint swollen, distended, painful Worse on movement	
Ledum	Injured joint cold and numb, Much swelling	
Rhus toxicodendron	After *Arnica* Hot, swollen, painful joint, creaky on first movement; better when limbs up	

SPRAINS

Remedies	General Indications	First-Aid Measures
Ruta graveolens	Torn and wrenched tendons or ligaments Bruised periosteum (bone covering), Worse in cold wet weather	
Symphytum (Internally and lotion)	After *Arnica* and *Ruta*, if necessary, Injury to tendons and the bone covering	

STRAINS

Remedies	General Indications	First-Aid Measures
Arnica	Sore, bruised feeling, Strained back muscles, Sore muscles	Elevate the injured part. Apply cold packs during the first 24 hours; heat after that. Wrap loosely with elastic bandage to support injured area.
Rhus toxicodendron	Sore muscles, Torn ligaments and tendons, Bruised periosteum (bone covering), Worse on first movement, better after limbs up	

WOUNDS

Remedies	General Indications and Benefits	Worse From	Better From
Arnica	Shock of injury, Speeds healing, Jagged wounds (internal use only)	Light touch, Heat, Rest	Head low
Calendula	Cleanses and speeds healing of : Abrasions (lotion), Scratches (lotion), Superficial wounds (lotion)	Lying on painful side, Slight touch, Slightest draft	Warmth
Hepar Sulphur	Red, swollen, painful wounds	Touch, Cold	Bending head backward
Hypericum	Relieves nerve pain and pain of jagged wounds, Cleanses and speeds healing of: Jagged, irregula cuts (lotion), Lacerations (lotion), Painful burns (lotion)		
Ledum	Cleanses puncture wounds (lotion)	Night, Heat of the bed, Warm applications	Cold applications

16

REMEDIES FOR INSECT'S BITES AND STINGS

INSECTS BITES AND STINGS

Remedies	General Indications and benefits	Worse From	Better From
Apis Bee for Hornet and Wasp Stings	Burning, stinging pains, Rapid rosy swelling, not bright red, Puffiness rather than hard swelling	Heat, Hot applications	
Arnica (Tincture) Bee for Hornet and Wasp Stings	Applied directly to the sting, relieves pain at once	Least touch, Rest	Lying down with head low
Calendula (Tincture) Bee for Hornet and Wasp Stings	Relieves pain and swelling when applied directly to sting		
Cantharis, Bee for Hornet and Wasp Stings	Red and inflamed stings, Burning sensation	Touch	Gentle massage
Carbolicum acidum for Poisonous Spider	Dusky red face, Pale around mouth and nose, Listless, sluggish Sensitive to odors		

INSECTS BITES AND STINGS

Remedies	General Indications	Worse From	Better From
Lachesis for Poisonous Spider, Scorpio and Snake Bites	Affected part dusky red or blue, Oozing of dark blood	After sleep	
Ledum (Internally or tincture) for Bee, Hornet, and Wasp Stings	Punctured wounds and stings, Numbness or high sensitiviy or high sensitivity to touch, Pains extend upward, Wounded parts may be cold	Night, Heat of the bed	Cold applications Cold bathing
Oxalicum acidum for Poisonous Spider, Scorpion, and Snake Bites	Affected part cold and numb Violent pain Trembling of hands and feet	Slightest touch Thinking about himself	

17

REMEDIES FOR BURNS

BURNS

Remedies	Instructions
Arnica	To be given first to prevent shock.
Cantharis	If pain persists after *Arnica,* give 2 tablets every 15 minutes until pain lessens. Repeat *Cantharis* if pain returns.
Causticum	If the pain is accompanied by restlessness and blister formation, give 2 tablets of *Causticum* every 15 minutes until pain lessens.
Aloe Vera	Gel from plant forms a protective covering, relieves pain and promotes healing.
Calendula Lotion	Immerse burned area in cold water with a few drops of *Calendula* succus or tincture. Saturate dressing with *Calendula* lotion to cleanse, relieve pain and heal.
OR Hypericum Lotion	Immerse burned area in cold *Hypericum* lotion. Dressing should be saturated with *Hypericum* lotion and applied to burned area to prevent serum loss and promote tissue formation.
OR Urtica urens Lotion	Soothing lotion when applied externally. Quickly relieves pain and heals. When older burns are characterized by itching and stinging, *Urtica* lotion relieves.

18

REMEDIES FOR SPORTS INJURIES

SPORTS INJURIES

Injury	Remedy	First-Aid Measures
Athlete's Foot	Calendula	Wash feet thoroughly with water and mild soap (preferably Calendula soap). Apply Calendula ointment. Expose feet to air. Avoid synthetic or colored hose.
Bleeding from mouth	Calendula	Rinse mouth with Calendula lotion.
Blisters Raw burning pains; Better from cold applications	Cantharis	Clean area, bandage to protect from pressure and dirt.
Burning heat	Urtica	
Broken Rib Pain	Bryonia	Rest in comfortable position. Avoid jarring.
When pain lessens, To promote healing of bone	Symphytum	

SPORTS INJURIES

Injury	Remedy	First-Aid Measures
Bruises (Black eye, face bruise, heel or toe bruise, knee bruise barked skin, strains)	Arnica	Cleanse if necessary, Place ice pack over bruise.
Crushed Fingers and Toes	Hypericum	Rest and elevate injured part.
Cuts and Abrasions General	Calendula Lotion	Clean area gently but thoroughly with mild soap and water, rinse in clear water, then apply *Calendula* lotion. Apply a sterile, nonstick gauze dressing and leave it undisturbed. Keep dressing moistened with *Calendula* lotion.
Nerves (toes, fingers etc.)	Hypericum Lotion	Follow directions above, but substitute *Hypericum* lotion.
Fractures For shock and pain	Arnica	Keep patient warm and treat with *Arnica* to prevent shock. Apply ice to painful area. If victim with broken bone must be moved, improvise a splint to keep bones from moving.

SPORTS INJURIES

Injury	Remedy	First-Aid Measures
Jock Itch	Calendula Lotion or Ointment	Keep groin area clean and dry. Apply *Calendula* lotion or ointment. Use corn starch as dusting powder.
Nosebleed, Profuse bleeding from vigorous nose-blowing	Phosphorus	Sit quietly with head thrown forward. Pinch nostrils together for 5 to 10 minutes.
Bright red blood; gushing	Ipecac	If bleeding continues, pack nostril with plug or sterile gauze. Lie down on your back with head elevated and cold wet cloth across face.
Overexertion Bruised sore feeling, Aching muscles and joints, General fatigue	Arnica	Rest followed by gentle exercise to limber up muscles. Warm, relaxing bath.
Shin Splints	*Arnica*	Apply ice pack to reduce pain; then heat treatment and gentle massage.
Sore Muscles	Arnica (Internally and lotion)	Externally, massage injured area with *Arnica* oil or lotion. Apply cold packs to ease pain; then heat.

SPORTS INJURIES

Injury	Remedy	First-Aid Measures
Sprained Ankle or Wrist if better from cold aplications	Ledum	Massage injured area gently with *Arnica* oil or lotion, but never on broken skin.
After swelling reduced	Arnica (Internally and lotion)	Elevate the injured part; apply cold pack during first 24 hours; heat after that.
After *Arnica*, if necessary	Ruta graveolens	Support injured joint with losely wrapped elastic bandage.
If weakness is still present after 2 weeks	Calcarea carbonica	Do as above.
Strained Muscles, Tendons, Ligaments	Rhus toxicodendron	Elevate the injured part; apply cold pack during first 24 hours, heat after that. Wrap injured area with elastic bandage for support.
Sunstroke and Heat Exhaustion, Face hot and flushed, Bursting headache, Waves of throbbing	Glonine	Move victim to cool or shady place. Put cold wet cloth on head. When conscious give one teaspoon of salt in a pint of water; encourage victim to drink several glasses.

SPORTS INJURIES

Injury	Remedy	First-Aid Measures
Pupils dilated, Pulse strong, pounding, Skin burning, dry flushed	Belladonna	
Nausea, Pallor, Clammy sweat, Prostration Pulse rapid and feeble	Veratrum album	
Cramping, in addition to *Veratrum album* symptoms	Cuprum metallicum	Wrap with elastic bandage to limit motion in painful joint.
Tendonitis (Inflamed tendon) Painful when begninning to move, better after continued motion, Worse in damp weather	Rhus toxicodendron	
Lame feeling, Lacks distinct characteristics of *Rhus tox.*	Ruta	

Contd...

Tennis Elbow	Ruta	Apply ice and rest the arm for a few days. Apply cold pack during first 24 hours, heat after that.
Twisted Knee		
Take on first day	Arnica	Wrap the injured part to limit motion.
If worse from slightest motion; take on second day	Bryonia	Elevate and rest the injured knee.

19

REMEDIES FOR EMERGENCIES

REMEDIES FOR EMERGENCIES

Remedy	General Indications	Worse From	Better From
Aconite	To diminish inflamation,	Night	Open air
For every Injury	To relieve pain	Warm room	
For Conditions with fever	Sudden onset, Restless, Fearful	Lying on painful side	
Apis mellifica For Breathing difficulty	Allergic shock, Reactions to bee stings, Throat passages closed, Tongue swollen	Heat, Touch, Hot applications Pressure	Motion, Cold bath, Open air
Antimonium tartaricum For Breathing difficulty	Cardiac fialure: drowning in own secretions Drowing, Cold and blue patient, respiration rattling, Respiratory failures, drowning in own secretion, clammy sweat	Evening Warmth Lying down at night	Sitting erect, Belching, Expectoration
Arnica For Bleeding	Caused by injury	Least touch	Lying down
For Eye injury	Black eye, Injury to socket, Soft tissue surrounding eye	Rest	Head low

REMEDIES FOR EMERGENCIES

Remedy	General Indications	Worse From	Better From
For Shock	From injury	After midnight, Cold	Warmth, Warm drinks
Arsenicum album For Asthma	Unable to lie down, afraid of suffocation, Wheezing respiration, Great debility, Burning in chest Worse from 1 to 2 A.M.		Head elevated
For Conditions with fever	Restles, Anxious, Burning pains, Thirsty for frequent small sips		Being semierect
For Food poisoning	Vomiting and diarrhea		
Belladonna For Conditions with fever	Sudden onser, Violent symptoms, Face flushed, Skin burning to the touch, Restless	Afternoon, Lying down, Touch, Jarring, Noise	
For Sunstroke	Pupils dilated, Pulse strong, pounding, Skin burning, dry flushed		Rest Quiet
Bryonia For Conditions with	Thirsty for large drinks, Skin pale, Irritable,	Motion, Touch	

REMEDIES FOR EMERGENCIES

Remedy	General Indications	Worse From	Better From
Fever	Desires quiet	Warmth	
Calendula (lotion) For Eye injury	Control of bleeding		
Carbo vegetabilis For Asthma	Onset after long spasmodic coughing spell with gagging and vomiting, Sore raw chest with difficult breathing, especially in evening, Air hunger, must be fanned, Bluish face, cold breath, Symptoms worse after eating or talking	Evening, Open air, Wine Warm, damp weather	Belching Fanning
For Bleeding, External or Internal	Dark blood, steady oozing		
For Collapse	From any cause, Air hunger, Cold breath, Sweat, cold and clammy		
Chamomilla For Fainting	From severe pain	Night, Open air, Heat	Being carried, Warm wet weather

REMEDIES FOR EMERGENCIES

Remedy	General Indications	Worse From	Better From
For Intolerance of pain	Air hunger (gasping for breath), Faintness, Ringing in ears, Dimming of vision	Anger	
China For blood loss resulting in:	With weakness and any of the above	Slightest touch, Draft, After eating, Loss of vital fluids	Hard pressure, Open air, Warmth
For After effects of loss of any vital fluids	From excitement		
Coffea For Fainting For Sleeplessness	From excitement or joy	Excessive emotions, Strong odors, Noise, Open air, Cold	Warmth, Lying down, Holding ice in mouth
Cuprum metallicum For Heat exhaustion	Cramping in addition to *Veratrum album* symptoms	Contact, Vomiting	Perspiring, Drinking cold water
Ferrum phosphoricum	Red cheeks, Gradual onset	Right side, Night 4 to 6 A.M.	Cold applications

REMEDIES FOR EMERGENCIES

Remedy	General Indications	Worse From	Better From
For Conditions with fever	Soft and rapid pulse	Touch, Jar, Motion	
Gelsemium For Condition with fever	Aching, Chilly Drooping eyes	Excitement, Damp weather	Open air, Continued motion, Profuse urination
For Influenza	Lethargic	Left side, 6 A.M. to noon Motion, Jarring, Stooping, Lying down	Brandy
Glonine For Sunstroke	Face hot and flushed, Bursting headache, Waves of throbbing, Skin sweaty		
Hepar sulphur For Fainting	From slight pain	Dry, cold weather	Warmth, After eating Damp weather
Hypericum For Eye injury	Excessive and long-lasting pain, Pain after removal of foreign object (lotion as an eyewash)	Cold, Touch	Bending head backward

REMEDIES FOR EMERGENCIES

Remedy	General Indications	Worse From	Better From
Ipecacuanha For Asthma	Sudden onset, Wheezing, gasps for air, Must sit up to breathe, Violent, rattling cough with every breath, Unable to bring up any mucus, Suffocates and gags with cough, Feeling of weight on chest	Moist, warm wind Lying down	Cold applications
For Bleeding	Bright red blood, Gushing, Gasping for air, Nosebleed, Severe nausea, Weak pulse, Cold sweat		
Ledum For Eye injury (internally and lotion)	For pain after *Arnica* fails to relieve	Night, Heat of the bed	
Nux vomica For Asthma	Attack often follows stomach upset with much belching, Oppressed breathing with shallow respiration, Tight, dry, hacking cough, Cough brings on bursting headache, Irritable, Hypersensitive	Morning, Mental exertion, After eating, Touch Dry weather, Cold	Evening, Uninterrupted nap, Damp wet weather, Strong pressure

REMEDIES FOR EMERGENCIES

Remedy	General Indications	Worse From	Better From
Phosphorus For Bleeding	Profuse bleeding anywhere, Nosebleed: profuse or from vigorous blowing	Twilight, Lying on left or painful side	Lying on right side, Dark, Cold
For Conditions with fever	Thirst for cold drinks, Appears well despite high temperature, Cold travel to chest, Cough, Sweats at night	Touch, Physical or mental exertion, Warm food or drink, Getting wet in hot weather, Ascending stairs	Cold food, Open air, Sleep, Washing in cold water
Pulsatilla For Fainting	From hot, stuffy atmosphere	Heat, After eating	Open air, Motion, Cold applications
Pyrogen For Conditions with fever	Aching, Pulse and temperature out of proportion, Restless, bed feels too hard		Motion
For Blood poisoning			
Ruta graveolens For Eye injury	Eye-strain followed by headache Painful, red, hot eyes	Lying down Cold, wet weather	

REMEDIES FOR EMERGENCIES

Remedy	General Indications	Worse From	Better From
Sabina For Bleeding	Uterine hemorrhage	Least motion Heat, Warm air	Cool fresh air
Symphytum For Eye injury	Injury to eyeball, Pain in eye following a blow of blunt object		
Veratrum album For Heat exhaustion	Nausea, Pallor, Prostration, Pulse rapid and feeble, Clammy sweat, Weakness	Night, Wet, cold weather	Walking, Warmth

20

REMEDIES FOR A HAPPIER BABY

REMEDIES FOR A HAPPIER BABY

Remedy	Specific Indications	Guiding Symptoms	Worse From	Better From
Aconite For Colds	First stages of a cold Quickly Settles in chest Breathing sounds harsh	Symptoms come on suddenly, Onset after exposure to cold, dry winds Restlessness	Night, Warm Room, Lying on painful side	Open air
For Group	Hoarse, dry, croupy cough, Loud, difficult breathing, Grasps throat with cough	anxiety; fear		
For Diarrhe	Watery stools, Crying; sleepless; restless			
For Ear infections	Swollen, hot, red, painful external ear			
For Vomiting	From nervous upset or fright, Profuse sweat increased urination			

Contd...

REMEDY	SPECIFIC INDECATION	GUIDING SYMPTOMS	WORSE FROM	BETTER FROM
For Diarrhea	Frequent, dark, offensive stools, After eating and drinking	Thirsty for frequent small sips, Burning pains	Eating and drinking, Cold Seashore	Drinks
For vomiting	From spoiled food, too much fruit, After eating and drinking, Nausea			
Belladonna For Colds		Sudden and violent onset, Restless	Afternoon, Lying down, Touch	Being semierect
For Ear	From getting head cold or wet, Generally right ear	Red face; hot, dry skin Feverish Eyes red; sensitive to light; pupils dilated	Jar Noise	

21

OBSERVATION: THE KEY TO PRESCRIBING

THE KEY TO PRESCRIBING

The essence of homoeopathy is building resistance, or stimulating the body's defense mech anism by selecting a remedy whose characteristics or "drug picture" matches the totality of the symptoms. The key to the choice of remedy is provided by the observation of those small differences that distinguish one person from another.

Two people "bitten" by the same bug may react differently, and therefore require different remedies. Take, for example, Jane and Dick, a couple who were exposed to a streptococcus infection at a party. Both became ill shortly after Jane was flushed, restless, burning with heat, thirstless, and acutely ill all of a sudden. Her throat was bright red, and her head pounded with each strong pulse beat. Jane needed *Belladonna* (deadly nightshade) for the strep infection. She took it and subsequently recovered rapidly. Dick was not so quick to show symptoms. He gradually became quieter, grew pale, and was very thirsty for large drinks of cold water, and wanted to lie perfectly still and be let alone; he was extremely irritable when questioned or disturbed. He developed a dry, racking cough. Dick needed *Bryonia* (white bryon), and, after taking a dose, felt better, apologized for his irritability, and was soon over his illness and back to work with no after effects.

If each had taken the other's remedy, that is, if Jane had taken *Bryonia* and Dick *Belladonna–a* highly unlikely situation because no homeopathic prescriber, even a beginner, could mistake these two remedy pictures–the "wrong" remedy would probably have had no effect at all. Jane and Dick might each have concluded, "I've tried homoeopathy and it doesn't work." This kind of reaction to homoeopathy occurs frequently; someone is treated with a homoeopathically *prepared* substance that was not homeopathically *applied* and, predictably, "nothing happens."

There is no such thing as an innately "homeopathic remedy." A remedy is homeopathic *only* when it is given for a condition whose symptoms match the symptoms of the "remedy picture," that is, the symptoms produced by the remedy when "proven" by a healthy subject. A wrong remedy is never homeopathic to the illness. Only the remedy which is homoeopathic to the illness can produce the desired result.

To be a good prescriber, that is, to find the remedy to match the symptoms of the ill person, you must be alert for those individual symptoms we call "rare and peculiar." You can train yourself to be a good observer by learning what to observe. If you've taken care of a small child, then you have already learned to be aware of the non-verbal expressions that signify discomfort, likes, and dislikes. An ill person of any age may not feel like making the effort to answer questions, so use your eyes, ears, nose, your sense of touch-observe!

Here is an Observation Checklist for the home prescriber. Knowing what to look for will make it easier or match the symptoms of the patient to the remedy. After you've used this Observation Checklist a few times, the process will become almost second nature. Before attempting to prescribe, use all your senses and observe:

Color of skin–Is it pale, red, or circumscribed red?

Color of lips–Are they red or pale, dry or cracked?

Color of tongue–Is it red-tipped, red-streaked, white, or swollen? Is it dry or wet?

Expression–Is it anxious, frightened, stupefied, confused? Do the eyelids droop?

Position and movement—Is the patient quiet and still, lethargic or restless?

Mood–Is the patient irritable, nervous, angry, sad, or withdrawn?

State of mind–Is the patient irrational or delirious?

Skin–Is it dry, moist, clammy, hot, cool or cold, sensitive to touch?

Pulse-Is it rapid, slow, weak, or pounding?

How does the patient respond to touch-Does it hurt or comfort him?

Voice–Is it weak, hoarse, deep or husky?

Breathing–Is it gasping, rapid, difficult, wheezing, or irregular?

Speech–Is it incoherent, rushed, slow, or does the patient refuse to answer?

Where does it hurt? Determine the precise location of the pain. Ask the patient to point to painful spot with one finger.

At what time does the patient feel worse–morning, noon, afternoon, evening, or night? Before or after midnight?

What kind of pain is the patient experiencing? Is it aching, boring, bruised, burning or bursting, cramping, cutting or dull? Is the pain like a nail being driven in, or is it pressing' or stitching?

What are the patient's physical wants? Does he crave fresh air? Does he ask for cold or hot drinks? Does he like cold applications or warm ones? Does he feel better in general from warmth or from cold?

How does he smell-sick, sour, sweet, musty or offensive?

For example, your husband, Jack, comes home complaining of a headache and doesn't want any dinner. He goes to bed at once and asks for an extra blanket. He had seemed fine when he left this morning, but now his temperature registers 102 degrees farenheit; he is chilly, beginning to ache all over and can't seem to get warm. When you look in on him, he appears to be asleep but, on closer look, you see he is awake with drooping eyelids. You offer him a drink of water that he refuses.

Making your observations according to the Observation Checklist, you note that his face appears flushed, with dry lips, and his expression dull and stupefied. He is quiet and lethargic and wants to be let alone. He becomes irritable only when you persist in questioning him. Touching him, you find his skin is hot and dry; although he complains of feeling chilly. He has a slightly sour or sickish odor. When you ask him about his headache, he replies in a weak voice that it's a dull aching pressure like a band around his head.

Even given the right remedy, speed of recovery will vary from person to person. One may recover overnight, provided that he has a strong defense mechanism, or what we call a "good constitution." On the other hand, he may not be so fortunate. Perhaps he has inherited a tendency toward diabetes and his health is further affected by living in a city that has a high pollution index. In addition, he works in an office in which several people smoke, further polluting his air space. Under these circumstances, one may take several days to recover, but he will do so in less time than he would if he dosed himself with patent medicines that suppress symptoms rather than assist the defense mechanism.

Make a habit of keeping a notebook in which you note down symptoms of each family member during an illness. Besides helping you as a prescriber, the notebook will serve as a record of the course of the illness and, over a period of time, show the patterns of illness in the family and the most successful prescriptions.

If you live alone or are the only member of the family trained in homoeopathy, it is wise to familiarize yourself with the remedies and their indications while you're alert and well. In the event that you become acutely ill, if possible, write down all your symptoms. This will make it easier for you to be objective about your condition. Although it's nice to be looked after when you're sick, as a prescriber you have the advantage of knowing better than anyone else how you feel.